the joints of the ankle

the joints of the ankle

Verne T. Inman, M.D., Ph.D.

Professor Emeritus of Orthopaedic Surgery
University of California
San Francisco

The Williams & Wilkins Company
Baltimore

Made in the United States of America

Library of Congress Cataloging in Publication Data

Inman, Verne Thompson, 1905-
The joints of the ankle.

Bibliography: p.
Includes index
1. Ankle. I. Title.
QM549.I55 611'.718 75-38958
ISBN 0-683-04342-0

Composed and printed at the
Waverly Press, Inc.
Mt. Royal and Guilford Aves.
Baltimore, Md. 21202, U.S.A.

foreword

A preliminary draft of this monograph was submitted to me with a request from the author for my evaluation and reactions to its possible publication. I was flattered by this request, and after reading the text and receiving a favorable report from Dr. Ernest Gardner, Professor of Neurology, Orthopaedic Surgery, and Anatomy at the University of California, Davis, I encouraged Dr. Inman to submit the material promptly for publication. I am happy that Williams & Wilkins has accepted the book and has expedited its publication.

Verne T. Inman, a recipient of the Ph.D. degree in anatomy in addition to the M.D. degree, is also well versed in bioengineering. He is Emeritus Professor of Orthopaedic Surgery at the University of California, San Francisco, and was Director of the Biomechanics Laboratory at the same institution from 1957 to 1973. He is one of the very few orthopaedists who has the background and knowledge to write authoritatively about biomechanical subjects. This outstanding monograph is based on detailed and carefully executed morphological and biomechanical studies of the talocrural joint, the tibiofibular syndesmosis, and the subtalar joint. It explains their structure and function based on determination of axes by means of various mechanical devices. Throughout, Dr. Inman has used carefully and thoughtfully devised concepts and determinants, which are ingenious and always sound.

This beautifully reasoned and organized book is a culmination of twenty years of interest and study. Although at first perusal the methods used for analysis may appear to be complex, it soon becomes evident that this is not the case. They can be easily understood, not only by biomechanically oriented engineers, but also by students, residents, and practitioners of medicine interested in the subject, and by others involved in the care of patients with locomotor disturbances.

Dr. Inman's earlier publications concerning the intervertebral disk, the function of the shoulder joint and clavicle, the function of the hip, and the major determinants in normal and pathological gait are classics in their field. *The Joints of the Ankle* will, I believe, be accorded similar acclaim.

I was honored to be asked by the author to write this foreword, and it has been a privilege to do so. It has been comparatively recently that the principles of physics and engineering have been applied to the investigation of gait and posture, and Dr. Inman has been the leader of the small band of scientists in this field. This book was produced by the master of this group and assuredly deserves success.

Paul R. Lipscomb, M.D.
Professor of Orthopaedic Surgery
University of California, Davis

preface

This study was initiated by a simple desire to be able to align the axis of a short leg brace accurately with the anatomic axis of the ankle joint. Originally it was assumed that sufficient information could be obtained from standard textbooks of anatomy and pertinent articles in the literature to provide a clear definition of this axis, after which methods of locating it in the living could be readily devised. This assumption proved to be wishful thinking. The textbooks of anatomy are vague in their description and often actually contradictory. Specific articles in the orthopaedic and anatomic literature not only failed to provide the information desired, but led to utter confusion. Some authors indicated that the talus rotates within the mortise about a single axis, while others offered evidence that appeared to prove that a single fixed axis of rotation is impossible and that the axis must therefore be a continually changing one. Others pointed out that the axis is obliquely oriented to the joint surfaces, while still others seemed to assume that the axis parallels the joint surfaces. None of the textbooks related the axis quantitatively to easily palpable bony structures about the ankle which could be utilized in the living to approximate the axis, whether fixed or moving.

Although the original intent of this monograph was to report studies limited solely to the ankle (talocrural) joint, a search for a satisfactory explanation for the peculiar disposition of the calcaneofibular ligament necessitated that certain investigations on the subtalar joint be initiated. As these studies progressed, it became more and more apparent that the statements in the literature are also confusing and the reported observations required confirmation; thus there was a need for adequate anthropometric studies. Furthermore, it soon became clear that there exists an interrelationship between the talocrural and talocalcaneal joints that is so close that one cannot investigate one and neglect the other. An explanation for the anatomic arrangement of specific ligamentous structures, an understanding of the observed variations in the contributions of the two joints to locomotion, and an interpretation of certain clinical observations are only possible when one considers both of these articulations as a single functioning unit. An appreciation of the existence of this close functional relationship is indicated in the German literature, where the ankle (talocrural) joint is called the upper ankle joint (*oberes Sprunggelenk*) and the subtalar (talocalcaneal) joint is called the lower ankle joint (*unteres Sprunggelenk*). When such a concept of a functional unit, comprised of two interdependent articulations, is accepted, many puzzling facts become understandable and a whole new area is opened up for clinical research.

Acting upon an oft-repeated piece of advice of one of my revered professors, I decided to accept as true most of the quantitative data that were recorded in the literature, but to reevaluate the conclusions of the authors. New and different explanations would be sought. Early attempts to harmonize apparently discrepant reports revealed obvious gaps in the available data, so that additional investigations became necessary. Furthermore, many of the studies reported in the literature had been carried out on samples too small to evaluate adequately the effect of individual variation. Those few studies which appeared to be carefully carried out but on small samples were repeated on additional specimens before the published data were accepted as valid.

This report is a composite of many studies carried out over the past two decades by many individuals (students, residents in orthopaedic surgery, and members of the staff of the Biomechanics Laboratory), together with an exhaustive and critical review of the literature. At this time, credit and thanks should be given to many investigators who have provided valuable data. It is interesting to note that each author has reported his findings accurately. When his observations were repeated, they were found to be valid. Only the deductions as expressed by the authors have proved at times to be erroneous, apparently as a result of conclusions based upon too small a sample or a failure to consider additional factors that would have altered the interpretation of the findings.

This study has clarified a number of clinical observations that have been reported in the orthopaedic literature without adequate explanation. Several of these will be discussed in the light of newer concepts of ankle function.

In the following pages an attempt has been made to discuss the various aspects of the subject in a clear and simplistic manner. The mechanisms that are depicted by the simple wooden models (see Chapters 10 and 11) may appear at first glance to be so unlike the actual anatomic parts that realism is lost. However, the models have been purposely simplified to emphasize functional relationships: extraneous anatomic details that might complicate the presentation are omitted. To achieve the necessary mental transition back and forth between model and actual anatomic structure requires an accurate knowledge of anatomy. During the reading of this monograph it is suggested that a good atlas of human anatomy be accessible and a disarticulated talus and calcaneus be available for manipulation.

The primary objective of this study has been an attempt to sort out the facts from the seemingly discrepant observations reported in the anatomic and clinical literature. To do so requires that these discrepancies be accurately identified; if, from the published data, the observations appeared to be valid, then the studies would be repeated for corroboration. Because the discrepancies are numerous, some categorical method is necessary for their presentation. This seems best done by considering various anatomic facts in a sequential and individual manner. Since a variety of discrepant conclusions about the ankle joint are based upon or seem to stem from observations and statements about the shapes of the trochlea of the talus and the mortise, this question is considered first.

VERNE T. INMAN, M.D., PH.D.

San Francisco

Acknowledgments

In 1945 work started on projects that were later to be consolidated into the Biomechanics Laboratory of the University of California. The first projects were established through the action of the Committee on Prosthetic Devices, which later became the Advisory Committee on Artificial Limbs, under the National Academy of Sciences, National Research Council. The personnel of these projects consisted of specialists in engineering and medicine. The charge given was to acquire basic information on human walking and to utilize this information in the design and development of improved prosthetic and orthotic devices. Continuing financial support has since come from the Veterans Administration, with additional funding at various times from a variety of sources such as the National Institutes of Health; the Rehabilitation Services Administration and its predecessors, the Office of Vocational Rehabilitation, the Vocational Rehabilitation Administration, and the Social and Rehabilitation Service; the Easter Seal Research Foundation; the Children's Bureau; the National Aeronautics and Space Administration; and the Orthopaedic Research and Education Foundation.

At the present time the information obtained over the past 30 years is being reviewed and prepared for publication in a monograph entitled "Human Walking." During the preparation of this monograph several areas that have been investigated by the Biomechanics Laboratory appeared to be peripheral to the main subject of human walking, but were felt to constitute valuable information that related indirectly to human locomotion in both normal and physically handicapped persons.

Therefore, a series of companion monographs constituting reference material are being written. The financial support for this monograph, "The Joints of the Ankle," was from a multitude of sources. The tedious labor of dissection of cadaver material and anthropometry was carried out by students under the Federal Work Study Program, in which the major costs were borne by the government. The Easter Seal Research Foundation, the Children's Bureau, and the Office of Vocational Rehabilitation also provided funds for the research involved. Support for editorial and stenographic assistance and for the art work was provided principally by the Social and Rehabilitation Service, for which many thanks are given.

I am greatly indebted to the following individuals for their enthusiastic and capable assistance and I wish to publicly express my sincere appreciation for their continuous interest and cooperation.

Jean C. Lieberman, Ph.D., principal editor for the Department of Orthopaedic Surgery and the Biomechanics Laboratory, was most generous of her time. Her ability as an editor is superb, including organizing material and checking multiple details in the manuscript. Her ability as a linguist assured me that my interpretations of the statements from the French and German literature were correct and the quotations were accurate.

Mr. Mark Mikulich must be given complete credit for all graphs, line drawings, half tones, and photographs. He demonstrated unusual insight into the problems of achieving the excellent photographs of the anatomic specimens and dissections, as well as those of apparatus, human subjects, and wooden models. I also wish to thank Ms. Irene Chramko, who assisted Mr. Mikulich with the photography and who demonstrated a rare degree of patience in filing and cross-indexing the photographs and all reference material. I am grateful to Ms. Roxanne Tammik, who assisted in numerous ways in taking care of the miscellaneous details relating to the manuscript. In addition she acted as my personal secretary and cheerfully took care of a multitude of daily and extraneous chores, thus freeing me for writing.

contents

chapters

appendices

1

Shape of the Ankle Joint in the Horizontal Plane

WEDGE SHAPE OF THE TROCHLEA OF THE TALUS

The trochlea of the talus is generally considered to be wider anteriorly than it is posteriorly. Without exception, all texts on anatomy, if these dimensions are given, state clearly that the trochlea when viewed from above is wedge-shaped; its mediolateral transverse dimension is greater anteriorly than it is posteriorly (Horner, 1836; Gray, 1858, 1973; von Luschka, 1865; Quain, 1867; Hyrtl, 1873; Macalister, 1889; Testut, 1896; Charpy *et al.*, 1899; Fick, 1904; Rauber, 1906; Piersol, 1907; Frazer, 1933; Paturet, 1951; Sobotta, 1957; Rouvière, 1962; Bairati, 1963; Morris, 1966; Rauber-Kopsch, 1968; Gardner *et al.*, 1969; Grant, 1971).

Only in Cunningham's textbook (1964) is it stated that the "superior articular surface has almost parallel edges at the sides but the lateral edge . . . is bevelled . . . so that the trochlea appears to be considerably narrower at its posterior end," but elsewhere the wedge shape of the trochlea is recognized in a more positive manner: "In dorsiflexion, the broader, anterior part of the trochlea tali . . . ."

A few texts provide actual measurements for the differences in the transverse widths of the trochlea. Frazer states that the trochlea is about 4 mm wider in front than it is behind. Humphry (1858) and Piersol report that the trochlea is about one-fourth narrower behind than it is in front. Von Luschka states that the posterior end is about one-sixth narrower than is the opposite end. Fick reports an approximately 0.5-cm difference. Macalister states that the posterior width is four-fifths of the anterior width. Charpy *et al.* record: "*La différence de largeur en avant et en arrière est de 4 à 5 mm.*" Testut reports an anterior width that is from 5 to 6 mm greater than is the posterior.

Individual scientific articles that discuss the "wedging" of the trochlea also reveal similar discrepancies. Lane (1887-1888) states that, if the oblique facet for the posterior inferior transverse ligament of the tibiofibular syndesmosis on the lateral side is included in the measurement, the lateral and medial borders of the trochlea "run quite parallel" and never differ more than "about $\frac{1}{16}$ to $\frac{1}{19}$ of an inch." Sewell (1904), in an exhaustive study of over 1000 Egyptian skeletons from the Fifth Dynasty to the Roman period, reports that the average ratio of the anterior transverse dimension of the trochlea to the posterior transverse width is 1:0.8, with a range of 1:0.7 to 1:0.9.

Barnett and Napier (1952) investigated 152 cadaver tali and found considerable variation in individual tali, some showing marked and others minimal wedging. They expressed this variation by the "fraction 100 x/y." To compensate for the various sizes of tali, they apparently chose to express the wedging as a ratio, where x was the difference in width and y was the anteroposterior length (distance between the transverse measurements, which were taken perpendicular to the tibial facet). The implication of this variability is that individual tali may show parallelism between the planes of the tibial (medial) and fibular (lateral) facets while others show various degrees of posterior convergence of these planes. By calculation, the maximal angle of convergence in their series would be approximately 8° ($\tan^{-1} 0.14$).

The article by Barnett and Napier appears to be both a careful and an extensive study. Before their findings were accepted, it was thought proper to repeat their measurements in our laboratory on 100 cadaver tali. Their findings were completely confirmed. The only deviation was that in our series the "fraction 100 x/y" was found to vary between 0 and 19 rather than 0 and 14 as reported by these authors.

In addition, the average differences in the anterior and posterior widths of the tali were determined in our specimens (Appendix B). In each specimen the triangular (fibular) facet on the lateral side was included in the posterior transverse dimension to obviate the criticism raised by Lane. The average posterior width of the talus was less than the anterior width by 2.4 ± 1.3 mm, with a range from 0 to 6 mm. The distribution of these differences in widths is shown in the histogram (Fig. 1.1).

From the qualitative and quantitative information obtained from the literature, supplemented with measurements on 100 cadaver tali, the following conclusions seem clear and definitive. The differences in the anterior and posterior transverse dimensions of the trochlea range from 0 to 6 mm. In a small number of specimens (probably less than 5%) the sides of the trochlea are essentially parallel and no wedging is apparent. The vast majority of tali, however, show wedging of the trochlea; some tali show the posterior width to be as much as 25% less than the anterior width, or in absolute dimensions as much as 6 mm.

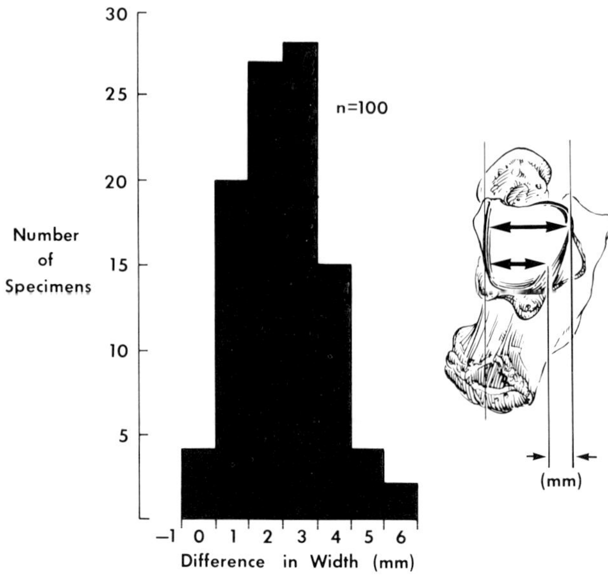

FIG. 1.1. Histogram showing distribution of differences in width of 100 cadaver tali. The measurements were made in a plane perpendicular to the surface of the tibial facet.

THE AMOUNT OF POSTERIOR CONVERGENCE OF THE MALLEOLAR FACETS

Consideration of the wedge shape of the trochlea of the talus in the transverse plane immediately raises the question of whether the malleolar facets are oriented so as to parallel the corresponding articular surfaces on the medial and lateral sides of the trochlea. If so, the planes of the malleolar facets should also converge posteriorly. This is implied in the majority of textbooks of anatomy by such remarks as the "malleoli tightly embrace the talus in all positions of the joint" (Gray, 1973) or by the reproduction of drawings of the mortise showing the convergence of the malleoli but without exact statements in the text. Only a few texts specifically state that the distance between the articular surfaces of the malleoli is greater anteriorly than posteriorly (Fick, 1904; Bairati, 1963; Cunningham, 1964), while only two give quantitative data and state that the anterior and posterior malleolar distances vary from 4 to 5 mm (Charpy *et al.*, 1899; Frazer, 1933).

No other specific works in the anatomic and orthopaedic literature were discovered that supplied measurements on the amount of posterior convergence of the malleolar facets.

To supplement the meager information available in the literature and to confirm the impression that the planes of the malleolar facets do converge posteriorly and therefore conform to the tibial and fibular facets of the talus, the following observations were made. One hundred dissected cadaver ankle joints were carefully inspected. In all cases the contiguous articular surfaces between malleolar and talar facets appeared to remain in contact during the entire range of ankle motion, indicating that parallelism between articulating surfaces was maintained. To confirm this visual impression, the angles of convergence between the planes of the facets were measured separately on each talus and on the corresponding cast of the interior of each mortise. For the casts, dental stone, which demonstrates no shrinkage on setting (actually there is 0.9% expansion), was used (Appendix A).

On each specimen, the angle of posterior convergence of the lateral facets of the talus and the corresponding angle of the malleolar facets were found to be identical. This fit between mortise and trochlea is well expressed by Humphry (1858) when he states, "The upper articular surface of the astragalus is one-fourth wider in front than behind; the cavity between the tibia and fibula, into which it is received, is shaped in a corresponding manner."

2

The Axis of the Ankle Joint

MISCONCEPTIONS PROMULGATED IN THE LITERATURE

Almost without exception, textbooks of anatomy describe the ankle joint as a typical hinge joint (ginglymus). Although rarely specifically stated, it is implied that rotation of the talus within the mortise is about a single axis. The location of this axis is never accurately defined, but either by direct statement or by inference it is considered to be horizontal (or, in one case, nearly horizontal—see the statement below by Testut and Latarjet (1948)) and to parallel the articular surfaces of the joint. The vague descriptions are amplified in a few textbooks by the addition of such details as the following. The axis passes through the tip of the lateral and slightly below the medial malleolus (Cunningham, 1964); the axis passes approximately through the end of the outer malleolus, and below and behind the inner malleolus (Frazer, 1933); the horizontal, transverse axis passes through the talus beneath the tip of the medial malleolus (Rauber-Kopsch, 1968); the horizontal axis passes below the most distal tip of the medial malleolus, runs through the talus, and passes through the outermost prominence of the lateral malleolus (Braus, 1954); the axis passes through both malleoli (Benninghoff and Goerttler, 1960; Gardner *et al.*, 1969); a transverse axis that passes through the center of curvature of the trochlea but is not absolutely transverse but gently oblique from the inside to the outside and from front to back (Testut and Latarjet, 1948); a transverse axis drawn through the body of the talus (Morris, 1966); the transverse axis about which movement takes place is slightly oblique (Gray, 1973).

While there are differences in the horizontal direction of the axis of the ankle joint expressed in the various textbooks, they all essentially agree that the axis, when projected onto a coronal plane, is horizontal. The acceptance of this location is reflected in some recent clinical texts (Steindler, 1955; Cailliet, 1968), as well as in the Instructional Courses of the Twelfth Annual Assembly of the American Academy of Orthopaedic Surgeons: "the ankle-joint axis actually becomes oblique only in traumatic cases of malleolar fractures or in actual injuries to the epiphyseal plate of the tibia" (Steindler, 1952).

The assumption that a transverse axis paralleling the articular surfaces of the ankle joint exists has led anatomists and orthopaedic surgeons into a dilemma, for which an acceptable solution appears to have been reached more through armchair reasoning than through further investigation. The result has caused written explanations to appear which, in reality, are unsubstantiated by fact; they are both ingenious and at times somewhat amusing. The dilemma is easily stated: If there is a transverse axis, how can a wedge-shaped trochlea be accommodated during dorsiflexion into a mortise whose malleoli show a similar posterior convergence? This question was raised by Bromfeild (1773) when he stated that if the lateral malleolus were part of the tibia and no give or play whatever occurred between the malleoli, no one could take more than a very few steps without fracturing one or the other malleolus. The talus, however, does in fact rotate easily in the mortise, and several explanations are possible. One can ignore the anatomic facts and state that the wedge shape of the talus is only apparent and not real and so conveniently avoid the entire problem. This is done by Lane (1887-1888). Krause (1903) also evades the problem by stating that the trochlea rotates about a vertical axis located within the fibula during flexion and extension of the ankle and therefore does not actually need to force open the mortise.

If a transverse axis is assumed, acceptance of the wedge-shaped trochlea into the wedge-shaped slot formed by the malleoli can be explained by only one of two reasonable alternatives. Either the distance between the malleoli must change during movement of the ankle, or the malleoli remain stationary and the ankle becomes tight on dorsiflexion and lax on plantar flexion. These explanations, either individually or in combination, are stated in all textbooks of anatomy that were available for review.

SEPARATION OF THE MALLEOLI

Having assumed that movement of the fibula constitutes the essential mechanism by which the mortise adjusts to the varying widths of the trochlea, most writers of textbooks have accepted any slight movement in the tibiofibular syndesmosis as adequate confirmation. Few investigators seem to have actually calculated or measured the amount of movement of the fibula that may be necessary to accommodate for the degree of wedging of the trochlea. The earliest were Ashhurst and Bromer (1922), who say they "have measured it [separation of malleoli] by affixing a wire in each malleolus and bending the ends of these wires forward over the ankle joint until they crossed each other: . . . by scratching a mark on each wire at the same point when the foot is in full plantar flexion, it is easy to measure the excursion as the foot is brought up into full dorsiflexion. This excursion, which exceeds two mm . . . allows the wider anterior diameter of the articular surface of the astragalus to pass back between the malleoli in dorsiflexion."

This method of measuring malleolar separation was ingenious, and it is certain that the amount of movement between the wires did occur as described. However, two criticisms can immediately be stated; one concerns the technique and the other relates to the conclusions. The separation of the marks on the parallel wires would also occur through simple rotation of the fibula around a vertical axis, or, as these investigators assumed, by pure spatial separation in a transverse plane, or by any combination of the two. The conclusion as stated implies that the malleoli in all ankles separate by more than 2 mm on dorsiflexion.

The basis of this statement is not supported with any quantitative data. It is not known whether Ashhurst and Bromer investigated only one ankle or a number of ankles and, if the latter, whether this was the maximal amount of separation or an average. Furthermore, as we have seen above, the degree of wedging of the trochlea varies greatly and Barnett and Napier (1952) found no relationship between the degree of wedging and malleolar separation. Therefore the conclusion that this amount of separation of the malleoli is the sole mechanism that permits the ankle to dorsiflex remains questionable.

Most textbooks of anatomy carefully point out that the tibiofibular syndesmosis constitutes a very strong articulation between the distal tibia and fibula (Quain, 1867). Only a barely appreciable amount of movement is perceptible when the attempt is made to move this articulation in the embalmed cadaver, in the freshly amputated leg, or in the living at surgery. Wagner (1974) stated that some separation of the lateral malleolus from the tibia can be readily demonstrated during a Syme's amputation. After removal of the talus forceful manual pressure against the lateral malleolus causes the soft fat pad which occupies the interval between the malleolus and the tibia to be sucked upward into the syndesmosis. The amount of motion is estimated to be no more than 1 to 2 mm. To reconcile this demonstrable stability of the syndesmosis with the need for malleolar separation, several additional factors have been postulated.

Humphry (1858) stated that the "yielding of the outer malleolus in a lateral direction, under the pressure of the articular surface of the astragalus during flexion, and its recoil in extension, depend, not so much upon a yielding of the ligaments that bind it to the tibia, as upon the elasticity of the bone itself. Hence a careful examination will shew that, during flexion, when the malleolus is pressed outwards, the shaft of the fibula is, in its narrowest part, just above the ankle, bent a little inwards; and *vice versâ*, when the joint is extended, the shaft recoils to its former distance from the tibia." Winslow (1880) repeated Humphry's assertion.

If it were true that the bending of the fibula, "in its narrowest part, just above the ankle," were the mechanism involved in widening the mortise, one could reasonably expect that stress fractures would be likely to occur in athletes, joggers, and military personnel who subject the fibula to prolonged intermittent bending stresses. However, stress fractures occur less often in the fibula than in any other bone of the lower extremity. Of 700 stress fractures occurring in army troops, Morris and Blickenstaff (1967) found only five in the fibula (less than 1%). In 1948, Burrows reviewed all the stress fractures of the fibula reported to that date. Of the 91 cases, only 21 had occurred in the lower third of the fibula where the bending stresses have been postulated to be maximal. Griffiths (1952) reported eight cases in children ranging in age from 14 months to 8 years. All occurred in the lower third of the bone, but five were related to direct or indirect trauma to the fibula. These authors concluded that jumping appeared to be a more likely etiologic factor, in both adults and children, than merely walking or running.

Devas and Sweetnam (1956) reported 50 cases of stress fractures of the fibula. The authors further state that "stress fractures . . . occur most commonly from running on hard surfaces." Only two cases were reported from running on soft ground. The locations of the stress fractures are interesting and Figure 2.1 has been redrawn from the paper by Devas and Sweetnam. These authors felt that the etiologic factor in the production of stress fractures was the "strong recurrent and rhythmical contraction of the plantar and long toe flexors." Utilizing roentgenograms they were able to demonstrate "that powerful contraction of the flexor muscles approximates the fibula to the tibia." The repetitive bending of the fibula leads to fatigue of

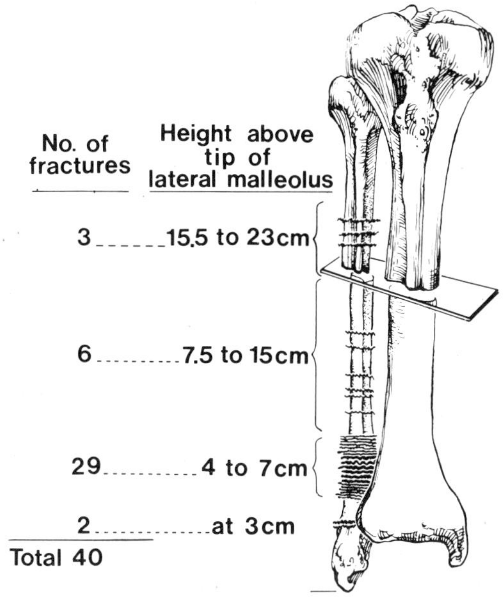

FIG. 2.1. Levels of stress fracture of fibula in 40 athletes. (Redrawn with permission, from Devas, M.B., and Sweetnam, R. Stress fractures of the fibula. *J. Bone Joint Surg.* 38-B:818, 1956)

the bone and fracture. The alternative possibility that the stress fractures might be due to wedging outward of the lateral malleolus with dorsiflexion of the ankle was not mentioned in the article.

Nancrede (1880) pointed out that "all the ligamentous fibres pursue an *oblique course from the tibia downward to the fibula*"; therefore a mechanism is provided which permits the fibula to move upward and outward or downward and inward, thus widening and narrowing the width of the mortise. While such a mechanism was postulated primarily on theoretical grounds and has not been supported by direct measurements, a modification of this concept has been accepted and promulgated in a recent textbook of anatomy (Grant, 1971).

In contrast to previously published reports, Weinert *et al.* (1973) and McMaster and Scranton (1975) stated that the fibula is displaced distally approximately 3 mm at the time of heel strike and during the weight-bearing phase. Such a displacement was measured by a high-speed camera on athletes during running with a skin marker over the lateral malleolus and by cineroentgenograms of the ankle throughout a full stride on an x-ray table. The method of measurement from "blow-up" prints of each frame of the motion picture film revealed the apparent distal movement of the fibula. However, the accuracy of such a measurement may legitimately be questioned. During the stance phase there are at least three different displacements that occur at the ankle joint: transverse rotations about the long axis of the leg, flexion and extension of the ankle (talocrural) joint about an axis that does not parallel the articular surfaces of the joint, and changes in inclination of the leg in the coronal plane.

The effects of possible differences in the profile projected onto the x-ray film are ignored. Before a distal displacement of the fibula can be accepted as an established fact, small radiopaque markers would have to be inserted into the tibia and fibula in the same coronal plane at the level of the tibiofibular syndesmosis.

A review of the literature obviously fails to answer satisfactorily the basic question of malleolar separation during dorsiflexion of the ankle. While perceptible movement of the fibular malleolus has been described by many authors, the only really quantitative data are those of Close and Inman (1952). These investigators inserted steel pins into the malleoli of 10 volunteers and with a dial indicator or, in one case, with a strain gage mounted on a strain ring, accurately measured the separation of the malleoli. Measurements were secured during normal walking and with full flexion and extension of the ankle during weight-bearing. The average amount of malleolar separation was reported to be 1.0 mm, with a minimum of 0.13 and a maximum of 1.8 mm. Close (1956) later repeated these measurements on 10 freshly amputated legs with essentially the same results.

If motion of the trochlea is conceived of as merely the insertion of a wedge between the malleoli, then some simple geometric calculations will demonstrate that the lateral malleolus must be displaced more than a just perceptible amount even though it is obvious that, because of the anteroposterior dimensions of the ankle mortise, any point on the articular surface of the mortise is not going to be displaced over the entire superior articular surface of the trochlea as the ankle joint is carried from full plantar flexion to full dorsiflexion. At most, this displacement probably covers not much more than half the entire articular surface of the trochlea. Therefore it is wrong to assume that the malleoli must separate to such an extent as to accept the total difference between the anterior and posterior widths of the trochlea. A better assumption would be to halve these differences. If this is done, then 1 mm of separation of the malleoli could conceivably accept an average talus; in cases of marked wedging, separation of 3 mm or more would be required.

However, even this amount of separation is never seen in anteroposterior x-rays of normal ankles, nor is it demonstrable in cadaver specimens, seen in the living ankle during surgery, or demonstrated by direct measurement. In addition, Barnett and Napier (1952) reported, "contrary to expectation," no relationship in their series between the degree of wedging and malleolar motion.

Fick (1904) expressed some reservations about the separation of the mortise, saying that it remains a question whether this conclusion is justified. At any rate, the concept of lateral malleolar movement as the complete explanation of compensation for the wedging of the trochlea is certainly inadequate, if not actually erroneous.

A further challenge to the unconditional acceptance of the notion that the fibular malleolus must be displaced laterally, rotate around its long axis, bend outward, or move upward in order to permit full dorsiflexion of the ankle began to appear in the reported clinical experiences of orthopaedic surgeons. Prior to 1930 the treatment for diastasis of the tibiofibular syndesmosis had consisted exclusively of externally applied compression and immobilization in plaster casts for relatively prolonged periods. The functional results of such treatment were often unsatisfactory, particularly in those cases in which complete reduction of the diastasis was impossible to achieve by external compression. Surgical exploration was undertaken and after adequate reconstitution of the normal relationship between fibula and tibia, the problem of holding the reduction became apparent. D'Aubigné and Smets (1934) reported their method of "*synthèse métallique*" in which a threaded pin was passed through the fibula and tibia and compression maintained by nuts threaded on each end. They reported, "*Dans tous les cas nous avons obtenu une correction parfaite du diastasis et un résultat fonctionnel excellent.*" The method was not immediately adopted by all surgeons. Alldredge (1940) recommended internal fixation of the fibula to the tibia by means of a screw or wire, but he was haunted by the fear of limitation of dorsiflexion, and stated: "Removal of the metal fixation should be carried out in every case as soon as the ruptured ligaments have healed. Failure to do so usually results in the loss of dorsiflexion because motions of the fibula are prevented when it is fixed to the tibia." In his article this statement was unsupported by any specific documentation.

The surprising finding that rigid internal fixation of the fibular malleolus to the tibia did not lead to limitation of motion or other disabilities of the ankle is nicely described by Meekison (1944): "I tried this procedure with some trepidation but was amazed at the universally good results it produced. Indeed, my second case was an English Sgt. Pilot, who made a trip to the Ruhr just seven weeks after operation." Lee and Horan (1948) stated, "Internal fixation is the best form of treatment." Outland (1943) employed a bone graft "driven into a drill hole in the tibia and fibula above the joint." In his discussion of Outland's paper Darrach volunteered that he had been "putting a bolt through the two malleoli." Costigan (1953) declared that "the safest and quickest method of reducing and maintaining a true diastasis . . . is by . . . internal fixation with an inch and three-quarter stainless steel screw." Furthermore Costigan, in reporting 25 cases, stated categorically that it was not necessary to remove the screw at a later date because of pain or diminished function. Mullins and Sallis (1958) reported 75 cases, in which the patients had an age range of 16 to 65 years, in which the tibiofibular syndesmosis was immobilized with a lag screw. "The results . . . have been uniformly successful."

In 1960, Grath published his excellent clinical and experimental study on the ankle mortise. This included an extensive and critical review of the literature and experimental measurements on the amount of tibiofibular separation in both cadaver and living ankles together with careful follow-up on 264 cases of ankle injuries treated operatively. Of these, 111 were treated by "transsyndesmotic fixation with a lag screw." In addition, Grath carefully evaluated 10 patients with a solid synostosis of the distal tibiofibular articulation. His conclusions may be summarized briefly. Little or no separation of the lateral malleolus could be demonstrated in the cadaver with lateral tensions of up to 40 kg or in the living lax ankle on dorsiflexion and plantar flexion. While some motion was usually perceptible it never exceeded a maximum of 2 mm. From his clinical studies he concluded that "*loss of mobility between the distal ends of the tibia and fibula does not by any means always lead to joint symptoms*" or to "restricted ankle joint mobility."

LOOSE FIT OF THE TROCHLEA IN THE MORTISE DURING PLANTAR FLEXION

Some editors of textbooks of anatomy seem to have appreciated that lateral malleolar separation alone is not an adequate explanation, so they choose to state that the trochlea fits snugly between the malleoli in dorsiflexion but that on plantar flexion, when the narrowest portion of the trochlea occupies the mortise, the joint is somewhat lax and lateral movement is permitted (Allen, 1882; Quain, 1892; Morris and Lond, 1893; Frazer, 1933, 1965; Paturet, 1951; Cunningham, 1964). This concept has also been accepted in the clinical literature (Lewin, 1941; Colonna, 1950; Howorth, 1952).

While many texts, especially modern ones, seem to accept without question the occurrence of increased lateral play of the talus within the mortise, some older investigators refute this. The following statement appears in the *Cyclopaedia-Anatomy and Physiology* (Todd, 1835–1836): "A slight degree of *lateral motion* of the ankle is perceptible in the dead subject, but during life it cannot be said to exist." Lane (1887-1888) emphasized that even in the cadaver "very little lateral movement can take place between the astragalus and the tibia and the fibula in the vigorous adult subject in any position of the ankle-joint." Only in Gray's *Anatomy of the Human Body* (1973) does this categorical statement appear: "The malleoli tightly embrace the talus in all positions of the joint, so that any slight degree of side-to-side movement which may exist is simply due to stretching of the ligaments of the talofibular (*sic*) syndesmosis, and slight bending of the body of the fibula."

Furthermore, a careful inspection of anteroposterior x-rays of the normal ankle taken in full extension and flexion never shows an increase in the distance between the lateral borders of the trochlea of the talus and the inner surfaces of the malleoli. Also, clinical examinations of the normal ankle always fail to demonstrate any perceptible lateral play of the talus in the mortise with full plantar flexion of the ankle.

This failure to perceive an increase in the lateral movement of the talus when the ankle is in full plantar flexion has led several authors to state that the collateral ligaments provide the necessary stability by becoming taut (Cunningham, 1905; Braus, 1954) and compensate for the supposed skeletal disparity between the posterior width of the trochlea and its mortise.

It is difficult to evaluate merely qualitative statements, but they can be interpreted in the light of available quantitative data. Some motion of the lateral malleolus can usually be perceived during motion of the ankle. This motion, however, is very small and appears to be insufficient to explain the acceptance of an average wedge-shaped trochlea into the mortise. Furthermore, there appears to be no support for the contention that there is an increase in lateral play of the trochlea within the mortise when the ankle is in full plantar flexion (particularly in the living individual). If these commonly expressed statements in the literature are either inadequate or erroneous, then there is a dire need for further studies and, it is hoped, a more satisfactory explanation will be developed which will fit the facts. A beginning can be made by reviewing certain suggestive observations which have appeared at irregular intervals in the literature.

THE INCLINATION OF THE ANKLE AXIS

The exact position of the axis of the ankle joint as projected onto a transverse plane is occasionally mentioned in textbooks of anatomy. Gray (1973) states, "The transverse axis . . . is slightly oblique." Cunningham (1905) states that the movements of the ankle "occur about an obliquely transverse axis, as is indicated by the natural outward pointing of the toes." Morris (1966) provides the following confusing statement: "In the normal position of the feet in standing, heels approximated, the two axes form an angle of about 130° open backward." Fick (1904), who felt that the axis of the ankle passes close to the malleoli, pointed out that the malleoli do not lie in the same coronal plane and stated: "*Bei 'sagittal' stehen-*

dem medialen Fussrand liegt die Spitze des lateralen Knöchels mit der des medialen in einer 'Frontalebene' oder ganz wenig dahinter." Only Paturet (1951) provides approximate measurements.

"*L'axe des mouvements est horizontal, mais non pas exactement transversal; il correspond à l'axe de la poulie astragalienne; oblique d'avant en arrière et de dedans en dehors, cet axe correspond approximativement à la pointe de la malléole péronière; de plus les mouvements de flexion et d'extension du pied ne se font pas dans un plan sagittal, mais suivant un plan vertical divergent en dehors et correspondant à l'angle d'écartement du pied de la ligne médiane* (25 *à* 30 *degrés*)."

Whereas the textbooks of anatomy have given little consideration to the position of the axis of the ankle in the transverse plane, the orthopaedic literature, while not extensive, contains pertinent information. The anteroposterior inclination of the axis as measured in the transverse plane has been termed "tibial torsion" by orthopaedists and "malleolar torsion" by podiatrists. Unfortunately most of the articles deal with the clinical interpretation of tibial torsion and the methods of treatment. The few that contain specific measurements have related the position of the ankle axis to the axis of the knee joint—only one relates it to the midline of the foot.

Le Damany (1909) appears to have been the first to report measurements on tibial torsion both in man and in animals. He employed a "*technique de la tropométrie du tibia.*" The midpoints on the two condylar surfaces of the tibia were located and a pin was inserted through the bone in line with these midpoints. The distal surface (plafond) of the tibia was divided midway between the anterior and posterior edges and another pin was inserted to parallel this line. The bony specimen was mounted vertically and the angle between the upper and lower pins was measured as projected onto a horizontal plane. Le Damany measured 100 right and 100 left adult isolated tibias. Fortunately he published individual observations so that it was possible to work with his data statistically. The average value was calculated to be 22° ± 10°, with a range from 0° to +56° of external torsion of the tibia.

Von Lanz and Wachsmuth (1938) reported no values for individual observations, but they did give ranges which indicated the existence of considerable individual variation. An average value of external torsion of the tibia was given as 23°, with a range of 7 to 48°. Hutter and Scott (1949), using a method of "tropometry" similar to Le Damany's, reported individual observations so that their data were available for analysis. The average value was 21° ± 10°, with a range of −4 to +40°.

The only other studies reporting quantitative data on tibial torsion were measurements made on children. These revealed a much greater variation in recorded values than in adults. Bergmann's (1962) report is an example. In his method the child sat on the edge of the table with the leg dependent and vertical. The angle between the edge of the table and a line connecting the two malleoli was measured. He reported over 1000 observations on two groups of school children. The first group consisted of 607 measurements on four-year-olds, and the second consisted of 601 measurements on ten-year-olds. His data, as published, divided the individual observations into separate groups, with each group containing all measurements that fell within 5° of each other. The data when plotted gave a normal distribution curve, indicating an adequate sample. His data were statistically analyzed; the average amount of external tibial torsion in the four-year-olds was −3.6° ± 9.5°, with a range of −25 to +20°. Among the ten-year-olds the average external tibial torsion was −1.6° ± 9.7°, with a range of −20 to +20°.

Swartling (1972) reported his observations on 150 unselected children (300 legs) ranging in age from one to six years. He employed a photographic method with the subject standing with knees extended on a barograph. Calipers fitted with rubber cups were clamped to the two malleoli and the femur at the femoral attachments of the collateral ligaments of the knee joint. Again, great individual variations in the extent of tibial torsion were found. Only a trend, similar to the observations of other investigators, was noted. This trend appeared to be an increase in the extent of external tibial torsion with increasing age. Among the six-year-olds the average angle was reported to be approximately 6.6° of external tibial torsion, with a range of −15 to +30°.

The only attempt to relate the position of the ankle axis in the transverse plane to the midline of the foot was made by Isman and Inman (1968). Observations were made on 46 adult cadaver specimens. Obviously the fixed position of the foot at the time of embalming influenced to a varying extent the relationship between the midline of the foot and the ankle axis, since the precise location of the midline of the foot was somewhat dependent on the position of the intrinsic joints of the foot. However, the measurements showed a greater consistency than did any of the studies which related the ankle axis to the knee axis. The average angle between the ankle axis and the midline of the foot was found to be 84° ± 7°, with a range of

69 to 99°. The inference that may be derived from the differences in the standard deviations is that the position of the axis of the ankle in the transverse plane is more constant in its relationship to the foot than it is to the axis of the knee.

It now appears to be definitely established that the mediolateral axis of the ankle deviates posteriorly from the coronal plane of the body to a varying extent. Nevertheless, the concept that this axis, when projected onto the coronal plane of the body, is horizontal and parallel to the articular surfaces of the ankle joint still persists. This erroneous concept of a horizontal axis of the ankle joint, which is expressed in nearly all standard texts, is not supported in any study which has been directed specifically toward the identification of the axis of the ankle joint, be it a single or a changing axis. The first specific statement that the axis of the ankle must be inclined to the joint surfaces was made by Golebiewski in 1894. In 1952 Barnett and Napier reported their findings on 152 cadaver specimens. The method employed by these investigators was an indirect one, based upon the determination of the center of curvature of the medial and lateral edges of the trochlea. Because the curvature of the medial facet of the trochlea was elliptical and not circular, they postulated that the axis could not be stationary but must be a changing one. However, they demonstrated unequivocally that the axis was not horizontal but was inclined "downwards and laterally" in relation to the joint surfaces. Hicks (1953), utilizing a method of minimal motion, determined the location of the axis of the ankle joint in 15 specimens. He reported confirmation of Barnett and Napier's findings. Attenborough (1966), by insertion of pins into the tibia and talus, demonstrated an angular change in the transverse plane of the leg with ankle motion, indicating that the axis of motion was obliquely placed. Isman and Inman (1968) investigated 46 cadaver ankles using optical methods of locating the points of minimal motion on the medial and lateral sides of the talus and subsequently articulating the talus within the mortise with a 3-mm rod to ascertain the accuracy of the axis while the joint was rotated through its entire range. These investigators found that in the coronal plane the axis never parallels the articular surfaces of the joint, but inclines downward from its medial to its lateral aspect, passing just distal to the tips of the malleoli as described by Barnett and Napier (1952).

While ample evidence has been presented by competent investigators to contradict the statements in anatomic textbooks that the axis of the ankle joint is horizontal, there still remains the need for more quantitative data to answer the question, does the talus move in the mortise about a single axis or is the axis a changing one? The concept of a changing axis of the ankle joint in flexion and extension is based upon the following reported observations. Barnett and Napier found that the contoured surface of the trochlea and its medial (tibial) side could not be fitted to an arc of a circle. Hicks, by the insertion of pins into the talus and malleoli of amputated legs, described a differing axis during flexion and extension. Sammarco *et al.* (1973) utilized a method of locating instantaneous centers of rotation from lateral x-rays of the ankle. The accuracy of the latter two studies is open to some question. Hicks (1953) used freshly amputated legs. "For experiments on the free foot the tibia was fixed to a support and movements were brought about by tensing or slackening the various tendons." It is conceivable that insufficient compressive forces were exerted by the individual tendons to force the articular surfaces of the ankle to remain in constant contact and this may have resulted in some undesirable laxness in the joint on movement. Unfortunately, in a later publication on the loaded living foot, Hicks (1954) does not again refer to his changing axes of flexion and extension. The accuracy of the results using the method of "instantaneous centers of rotation" depends upon the number and closeness of the points of least motion. The large increments employed by Sammarco *et al.* make their findings somewhat questionable.

The crucial questions requiring an answer are whether the axis of the ankle is a single stationary axis and if not, how closely it approximates a single axis, or whether it is a constantly changing axis and if so, what the limits of its variation are. To attempt to answer these questions a special apparatus was designed and constructed (see Appendix A for details of apparatus and procedures). The mortise of the ankle joint was inverted, with the tibia held firmly in a clamp and the fibula free. The isolated talus was securely fastened in a jig which was mounted so that it was free to move in all directions; at the same time a constant force was exerted perpendicular to the articulating surfaces. When the trochlea of the talus was articulated within the mortise, the motion of the joint was dictated solely by the curvature of the articulating surfaces. After the points of minimal motion had been optically located on the lateral and medial sides of the trochlea, a 3-mm stainless steel rod was passed through a drill hole through the talus, connecting the points of minimal motion. With the rod rigidly in place, motion of the talus in the mortise was examined.

It became immediately apparent that no rigid single axis could be established which would permit a full range of movement of the trochlea within the mortise while complete contact of all the articular surfaces of the mortise on the trochlea was maintained. Also, complete contact could not be maintained after removal of the restricting influence of the metal axis, with the talus rotated under load.

Since it was considered possible that changes had occurred in the articular surfaces as a result of the embalming, nine freshly amputated ankles were studied (without pins); the findings were the same. Only in the midposition of the joint was there apparently perfect congruity: On full plantar flexion 1 mm or more of separation occurred anteriorly between the mortise and the surface of the trochlea, while posterior separation occurred on full dorsiflexion. Although the articulating surfaces of the mortise and the trochlea are not matching components of a perfectly lapped joint, the degree of congruence is remarkably good. Simon (1971) measured the thickness of the articular cartilage in various joints in a variety of animals (bovine, canine, and human). He stated: "The elbow and ankle of the several species examined had thinner cartilage than other joints." In a later paper, Simon *et al.* (1973) reported on the degree of congruence under load in different canine joints. They stated that of all the joints in the lower extremity, the ankle, with the thinnest articular cartilage, demonstrated the greatest congruence: an average congruence ratio of over 90%. The conclusion expressed was that the ankle had fewer degrees of motion and that cartilage is thinner in regions of high congruence. The latter thesis was proposed in 1891 by Braune and Fischer. It appears that the ankle, while not a precision-machined joint, approaches this configuration more closely than any other joint in the lower extremity.

3

Fit of the Talus in the Mortise

Because the establishment of a rigid axis did not greatly alter the degree of incongruity of the surfaces or in any way alter the motion of the ankle joint, two additional studies were initiated. First, to determine whether the curvatures of the trochlea and the mortise are arcs of circles, the curvatures of each trochlea and its cast of the mortise were measured. Second, to determine whether incongruity between the mortise and the trochlear surface occurs at the extremes of dorsiflexion and plantar flexion, it was decided to study lateral arthrograms of a series of normal ankles.

CURVATURE OF THE TROCHLEA AS MEASURED ON ITS MEDIAL AND LATERAL SIDES

Barnett and Napier (1952) studied the curvature of the talus by projecting the fibular and tibial facets onto planes parallel to the surfaces of each facet. Since the planes of the tibial and fibular facets are not parallel, one or both of these can not be perpendicular to the empirically located axis of rotation. If the planes of the facets were obliquely oriented to the axis of movement, then obviously their projected curvatures could not be arcs of circles. This might account for Barnett and Napier's failure to fit the medial facet to an arc of a circle while they found the lateral facet to be such an arc. Since the carefully determined single axis in the present studies at least approximated a functional axis of the ankle, it was felt that all subsequent measurements should be related to this axis. Certainly, using the axis as the principal reference line for further anthropometric studies seemed more reasonable than selecting some arbitrary anatomic structure, plane, or line which might have no definite relationship to the motion of this joint.

Two sets of measurements were made on 104 cadaver ankles. Both were essentially intended to extend the observations of Barnett and Napier. The first set consisted of determining the angle, measured in a transverse plane, between the empirically determined axis of the ankle and the vertical planes of the fibular and tibial facets of the trochlea of the talus (see Appendix C). The second set was designed to determine the curvatures of the facets.

The angle between the plane of the fibular facet and the ankle axis was 89.2° ± 2.8°, with a range of 80 to 95°. The plane of the tibial facet was found to make an angle with the axis of 83.9° ± 5.2°, with a range of 70 to 93° (see Fig. 3.1).

The distribution curves for values on the two sides were distinctly different. When plotted, the angular values for the inclination of the plane of the fibular facet to the empirical axis of the ankle joint gave a normal distribution curve with a very narrow base (SD, 2.8°) clustered about a mean of approximately 90° (89.2°). The angles for the inclination of the tibial facet showed a much greater spread (SD, 5.2°) and a curve definitely skewed to the left (see Fig. 3.1). The coefficient of variation on the medial side (63%) was twice that on the lateral side (31%).

It is apparent that the plane of the fibular facet in all specimens always lies close to being perpendicular to the axis of motion. It is therefore not surprising that the curvature of the upper surface of the talus measured in the plane of this facet is an arc of a circle, as shown by Barnett and Napier.

The plane of the tibial facet is nearly always oblique

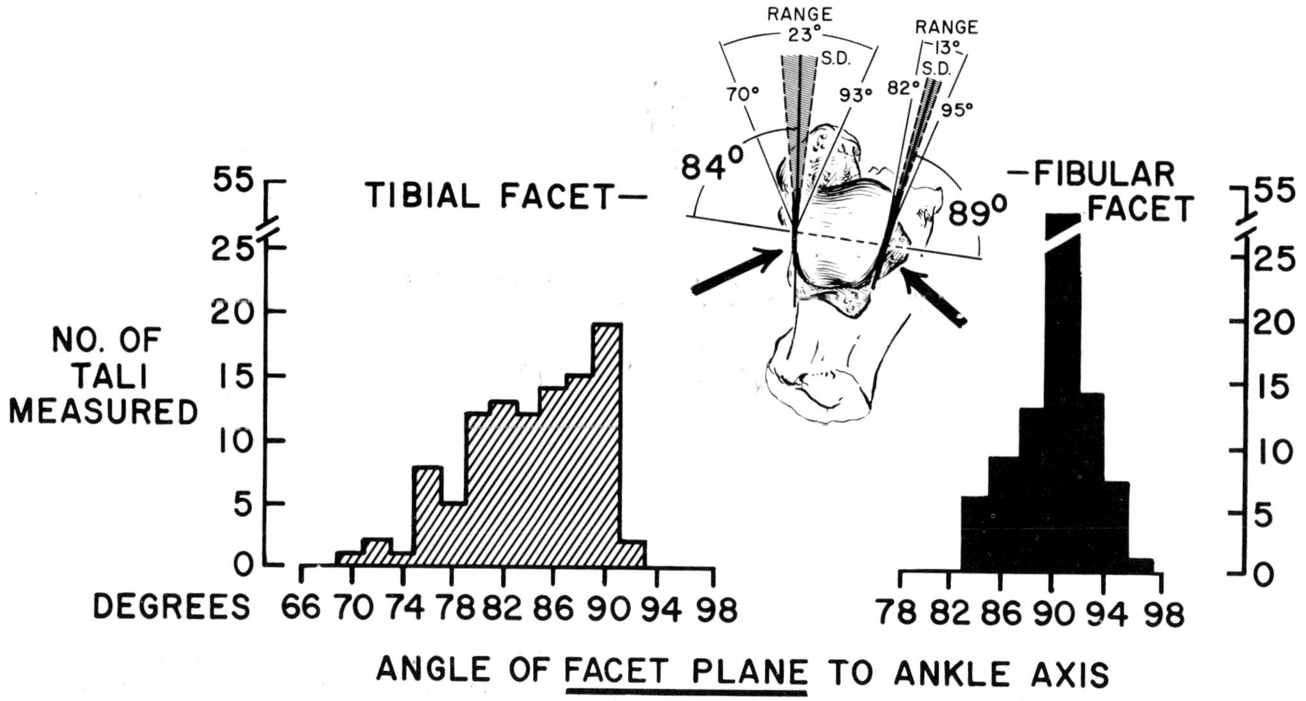

FIG. 3.1. Angle of orientation of tibial and fibular facets to empirical axis of ankle joint. The *histograms* depict the distributions of the values from 104 cadaver tali.

to the axis of the joint. Therefore, even though the surface of revolution of the trochlea may still be circular, its curvature when projected onto the oblique plane can not be an arc of a circle.

In order to determine whether the obliquity of the plane of the medial facet in relation to the axis of the joint is the complete and correct explanation for the failure of Barnett and Napier to demonstrate an arc of a circle on the medial side of the talus, it was necessary that the upper articular surface of the talus be contoured in planes always perpendicular to the axis of motion. Three independent techniques, using the following devices, were employed: a specially built contourometer, a Formagage, and a modified precision divider (see Appendix D).

In all tali the lateral side of the trochlea approximated an arc of a circle. This finding was in complete agreement with the published observations of Barnett and Napier. However, these authors state, "The medial profile . . . is compounded of the arcs of two circles of differing radii." In our series, where the surface of the trochlea was contoured in planes perpendicular to the empirical axis, we found that in 80% of the tali (86 of 107) the medial side of the trochlea was an arc of a circle, while in 20% (21 of 107) it deviated from an arc of a circle to a varying extent. Some deviated only the width of a pencil line while others had changing arcs of curvature whose radii differed by as much as 4 mm. The reason for this departure from circularity on the medial side in one of every five specimens is not clear at this time. However, it appears that in the majority of ankles the axis of the ankle joint can be considered for all practical purposes to be a single-axis joint. The fact that the plane of the tibial facet is usually oblique to the axis of the joint explains (for about 80%—see below) Barnett and Napier's finding that the contour of the articular surface of the trochlea in the plane of the tibial facet is never circular.

While the noncircularity was lessened by our method of direct contouring, it was not entirely eliminated in 20% of the tali, and the question of a "dorsiflexion" axis (the axis that obtains from the midposition of the ankle to full dorsiflexion) and a "plantar flexion" axis (obtaining from the midposition of the ankle to full plantar flexion), as postulated by Barnett and Napier from their method of contouring the trochlear surface, is only partly negated by our method of direct contouring about the empirical axis of the ankle. If the assumption is made that movement of the ankle must be related solely to the shape of the articular surface of the trochlea, then a changing axis must occur in these ankles. Barnett and Napier presented no quantitative data from which to calculate the possible angular change between their dorsiflexion and their plantar flexion axes. From the text of Hicks' publication (1953) a difference of 5 mm on the medial side can be estimated, and from his sketch a difference of 5° can be measured. These values agree with measurements of differences in radii of the medial trochlear surface in the 20% of our specimens which deviated most from true circularity.

Although it appears to have been recognized by all anatomists that the medial side of the trochlea possesses a greater curvature (smaller radius) than the lateral side, it is rarely so stated in the texts. However, the numerous drawings and reproductions in standard textbooks and atlases clearly depict this difference. Only Barnett and Napier (1952) explicitly state, "The anterior third of the medial profile is part of a circle whose radius is *less* than that of the lateral profile."

It was felt that this qualitative statement should be supplemented by measurements in order to determine the average difference and the degree of variability between individual specimens. Only the 86 tali that demonstrated circularity on their medial sides were measured.

Since the profiles of the articular surfaces on the two sides of the trochlea were available on the data cards obtained from the contour studies (see Appendix D), the following procedures were carried out. A chord was drawn from the farthest points of the articular surface on each side. Radii were dropped from the ends of the chords to the center of curvature. The lengths of the radii and the chords were measured to the closest millimeter. The chords were selected as an indicator of the extent of the articular surfaces on the medial and lateral sides of the trochlea rather than the attempt being made to measure the length of the arc. In addition the angle subtended by the enclosed arc between the two radii was measured to the closest degree.

The average length of the chords was found to be 21.4 ± 4.5 mm on the lateral side and 16.4 ± 3.8 mm on the medial side, indicating that the anteroposterior extent of the articular surface on the average was greater on the lateral than on the medial side. The length of the radii on the lateral side was greater in 77 tali, and in nine the radii were the same on the two sides. In no specimen was the medial greater than the lateral radius. The average difference in the lengths of the radii on the medial and lateral sides of the trochlea was 2.1 ± 1.1 mm, with a range of 0 to 6 mm. The subtended angles between the two radii on the medial and lateral sides, however, were almost identical, measuring 106° ± 13° on the lateral and 103° ± 14° on the medial side (Fig. 3.2).

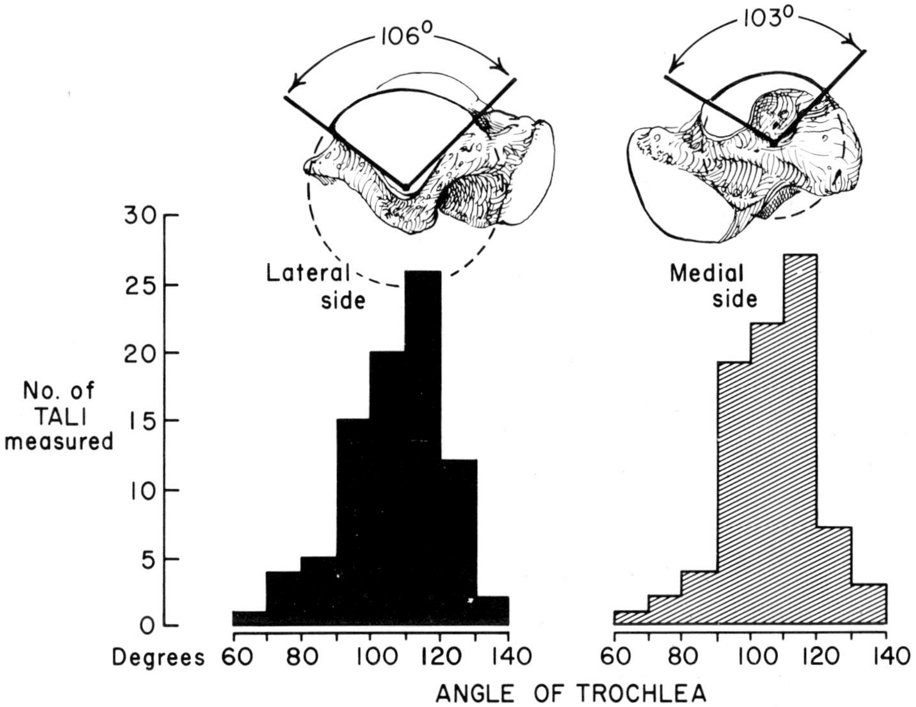

FIG. 3.2. Average angles, almost identical, subtended by arcs of curvature of trochlea on lateral and medial sides. Note that the distributions of the individual values as shown in the *histograms* are also similar.

COMPARISON OF ARCS OF THE FACETS WITH THOSE OF THE MALLEOLI

The trochlea constitutes only half of the ankle joint, and an investigation of the characteristics of the mortise is necessary to complete the study. Study of a concave surface, however, presents obvious obstacles to direct measurement; therefore, casts of dental stone were made of each mortise (Appendix A). These casts were used for further study, with the same techniques being employed as had been applied to the tali. Their curvatures were determined and the radii of curvature on the medial and lateral sides were measured (Appendix D). In addition, the medial and lateral anteroposterior dimensions of the articular surfaces were measured with the lengths of the chords as a basis.

The contour tracings of the malleolar facets of the casts of the mortises of 107 ankles (Appendix D) could in all instances be fitted to the arcs of circles. On the lateral side the arcs were always adequate in length, subtending an average angle of 69° ± 8°. This was sufficient to permit accurate fitting of the contour tracing to arcs of circles and to recognize readily any deviations from circularity. In all specimens the lateral side of the plafond was found to be circular.

The length of the arc of curvature on the medial side was always shorter than on the lateral side. The average subtended angle was 55° ± 11°. Those tracings which exhibited very short arcs (subtending angles of less than 40°) could often be fitted with several circles whose radii might vary by 2 to 3 mm. Therefore, it was impossible in approximately 15% of the casts to state categorically that the articular surface of the mortise on its medial side was truly circular or to be certain of the accuracy of the measured radii.

While congruity between the trochlea of the talus and its mortise on the lateral side of the ankle joint is a geometric possibility since both are arcs of circles of the same radius, on the medial side, in at least 15% of ankles, congruity has not been proved by this method and, furthermore, appears to be unlikely.

Since the radii of the arcs of curvature of each trochlea and of the cast of its corresponding mortise were available, these data were examined to determine the accuracy of fit between the trochlea and its mortise on both the lateral and medial sides of the joint.

On the lateral (fibular) side the arithmetic averages for the lengths of radii of curvature of the trochlea and its mortise as measured were found to be the same within 1 mm. When the data on each specimen were reviewed, it was noted that the radii for the trochlea and its mortise were recorded as the same in 30% (26 of 86), and in the remainder the radius of the trochlea was recorded as being either less or more than the radius of the mortise by 1 mm. Only in nine specimens was the radius of the mortise recorded as being 2 mm greater than that of the trochlea. The accuracy of measurement was not adequate to detect differences of less than 1 or 2 mm. From these data, however, it seems proper to deduce that the fit between the talus and its mortise on the lateral side is a close one.

On the medial side the difference in the measured radii of the trochlea and the mortise is greater. The average difference was 2.1 ± 1.1 mm, with a range of 0 to 5 mm; the radius of curvature of the mortise was longer than the radius of curvature of its trochlea in all specimens on the medial side.

One would surmise from these data that the talus fits snugly in the mortise on the lateral side, but rather loosely on the medial side. A few millimeters of anteroposterior displacement of the talus within the mortise on the medial side appears possible and such a motion could result in several degrees of horizontal rotation of the talus within the mortise.

Since this small disparity between the lengths of the radii on the medial side could be due to changes resulting from the embalming fluid or perhaps to technical and/or measuring errors, it was hoped that visual confirmation could be obtained from roentgenographic studies of normal ankles. However, since articular cartilage, which constitutes the true surfaces of contact, is not visible in routine x-rays, the study was made with arthrograms of the ankles. Attention was directed toward two possible observations. Could congruity between talus and mortise be demonstrated on the lateral side, as suggested by measured radii during a full range of movement, and could differences between medial and lateral sides of the ankle be detected?

ARTHROGRAPHY OF THE ANKLE JOINT

A review of published articles on arthrography of the ankle was made. It was not very productive; there were less than a dozen papers. In the majority of these reports, no mention was made of incongruity of joint surfaces. The x-ray reproductions of lateral views of the ankle were too often obscured by the opaque injection media to make it possible to identify the articular surfaces adequately. In those x-rays in which the articular surfaces could be clearly seen, the ankle joint was invariably in the neutral position (leg at a right angle to the foot). In these, the opaque medium was equally distributed between the articular surfaces, and the congruity between the talus and the mortise appeared to be excellent. Only Nagy (1965) shows x-rays with the ankle in full plantar flexion and dorsiflexion, and in these extreme positions some incongruity is readily discernible. In full plantar flexion the joint surfaces apparently separated anteriorly and on full dorsiflexion they diverged slightly posteriorly. These x-rays, however, were presumably taken while the patient was not bearing weight, so they can not be considered as absolute evidence of incongruity between the trochlea and its mortise.

Selected specimens from our anatomic collection were reviewed. They were articulated in the articulator (Appendix A) and the talus was rotated in its mortise, first free, and second, with the empirical axis fixed in place. In all specimens it was visually noted that in the midposition congruity between trochlea and mortise appeared to be excellent, while with plantar flexion and dorsiflexion from the neutral position various degrees of incongruity occurred. In full plantar flexion the posterior articular surfaces appeared to match well, but anteriorly there were varying degrees of separation. In full dorsiflexion the reverse was true. The incongruity appeared to be most marked on the medial side. While these observations tended to support the evidence obtained from the arthrograms published by Nagy, the visual inspection of the joint surfaces was limited to only a few millimeters of the anterior and posterior lips of the mortises.

It was therefore felt necessary to study arthrograms of normal ankles. To be adequate these x-rays must be true lateral views during weight-bearing in three positions: plantar flexion, neutral position, and dorsiflexion. Gordon (1970), in his series of arthrograms of 107 ankles, mentions the tilting of the mortise on the trochlea in flexion and extension of the ankle but without any statistical data as to frequency.

Dr. Gordon provided his 107 ankle arthrograms for review. Of these, 32 fulfilled the following criteria: The x-rays were true lateral projections; the contrast medium adequately filled the interval between trochlea and mortise and was clearly visible; and at least three views of the ankle were available, one in plantar flexion, one in dorsiflexion, and one in the midposition. Unfortunately only seven of the 32 were weight-bearing films. A study of these arthrograms led to several interesting observations.

In all instances a film of dye of an appreciable width was present between the articular surfaces in even the weight-bearing films. In the midposition, where the tibia was approximately at a right angle to the foot, there was good congruity in nearly all arthrograms. The width of the film of radiopaque dye remained the same from the anterior to the posterior edges of the plafond. In 13 arthrograms, good congruity was maintained in plantar flexion and dorsiflexion. In the remaining 19 persons the congruity was lost to a varying degree in plantar flexion or in dorsiflexion. The width of the film of dye became somewhat wedge-shaped, with the base of the wedge toward the center of the joint, and it was always more marked in dorsiflexion than in plantar flexion.

Two deductions seem justified from these limited observations. The articular surfaces never actually contacted each other, even in weight-bearing. A film of dye always occupied the interval between the cartilaginous surfaces. In nearly all the ankles, good congruity obtained only in the midposition. In this small series, over half of the specimens showed various amounts of wedging of the dye due either to rocking of the plafond on the trochlea, to rotation of the talus in its mortise, or to misalignment of the joint with the x-ray source. This occurred in both the weight-bearing and the non-weight-bearing films (Figs. 3.3 and 3.4).

The opacity of the dye to the x-ray made it impossible to determine whether the increase in the width of the dye film was uniform transversely across the joint or was limited to the medial or lateral side. Anteroposterior views were of little value in trying to answer this question since in plantar flexion and dorsiflexion the amount of dye within either the posterior or the anterior compartment of the capsule obscured the precise region that was of interest. Further studies with a less radiopaque material would be desirable.

The failure to demonstrate by anthropometry true circularity of the surface of the trochlea on its medial side in 20% of the specimens and the failure to show uniform contact between the joint surfaces by arthrography in a small series seems to indicate that all ankles can not be considered to move through single axes. However, the interesting fact remains that the available data indicate that the majority of ankles do rotate about axes which for practical purposes can be considered single and fixed.

On the other hand, the finding that an appreciable number of ankles may move through changing axes because of noncircularity of the medial side of the trochlea, because of loose fit of the trochlea in its mortise, or because of rocking of the plafond on the

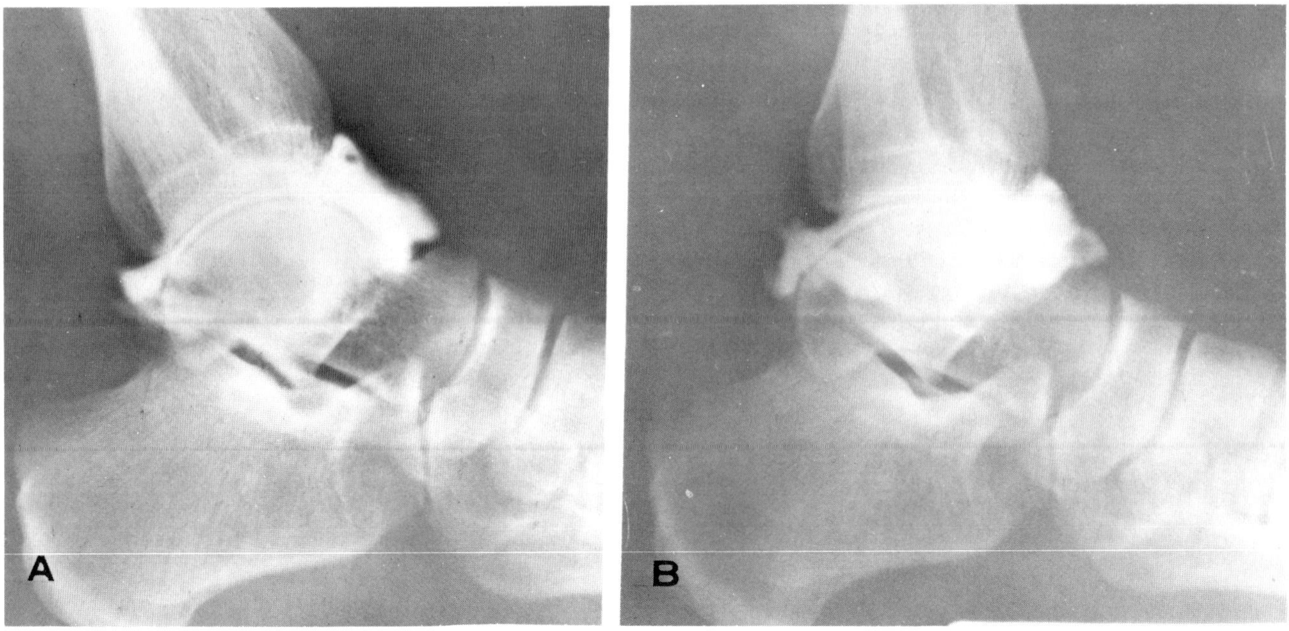

FIG. 3.3. Weight-bearing arthrograms of ankle. Note good congruity as revealed by the constant width of the dye column in plantar flexion (*A*), with wedging of the dye shadow in the midposition (*B*). (Courtesy of Dr. Robert B. Gordon)

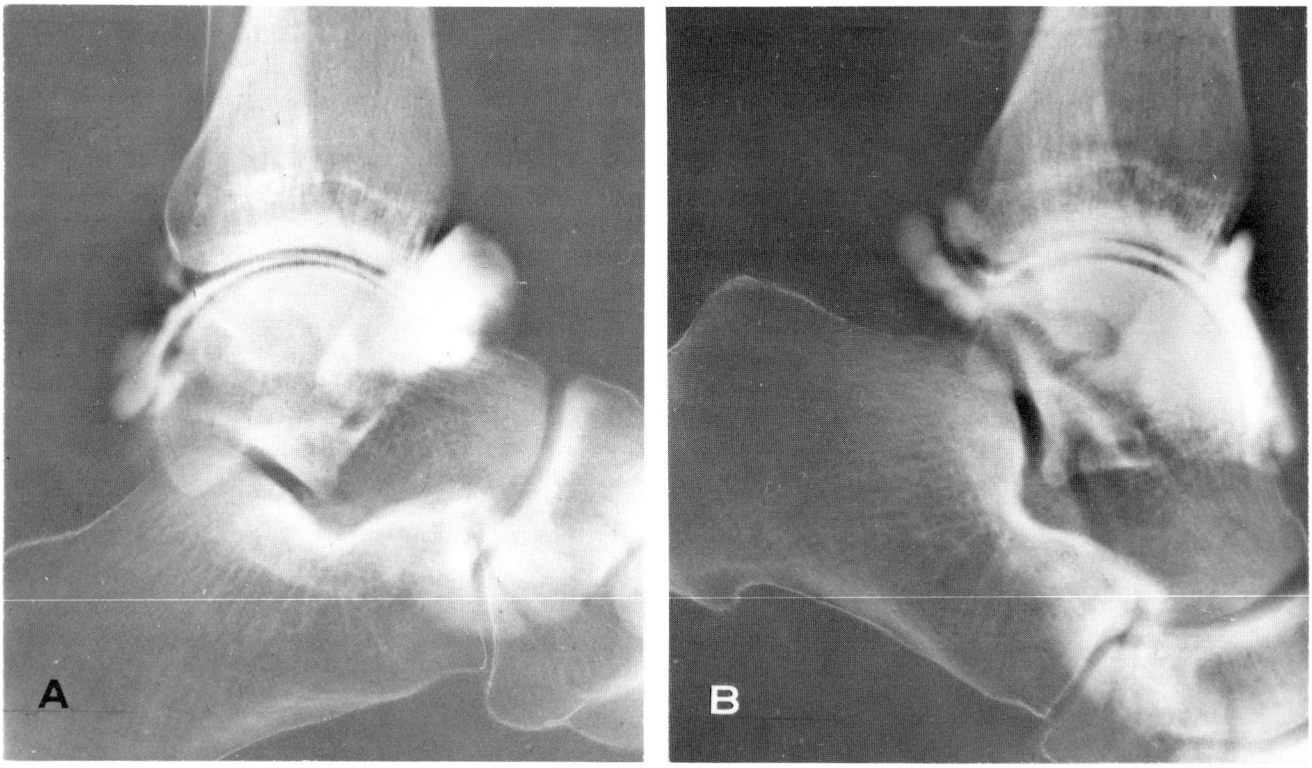

FIG. 3.4. Non-weight-bearing arthrograms of ankle in slight dorsiflexion (*A*) and plantar flexion (*B*). Note the minimal wedging of the dye shadow in dorsiflexion. (Courtesy of Dr. Robert B. Gordon)

trochlea, should not be discarded as possible technical errors or annoying deviations from normality. Instead, these characteristics may reflect functional adaptations and may prove to be clinically significant. Certain indications that this may be so will be discussed in a later section. At present, however, attention must be refocused on the main objective of this study, which is to attempt to harmonize the various apparently discrepant statements in the literature. This is best done by summarizing our present information.

4

Recapitulation of Observations

In the light of the preceding material, the following summary statements of findings and conclusions may be made.

1. The trochlea of the talus, viewed from above, shows various degrees of wedging from individual to individual. The degree of the wedging may vary from no wedging (± 5%) to marked wedging (the posterior width may be 25%, or as much as 6 mm, less than the anterior width).
2. The malleoli show a similar convergence posteriorly.
3. The articular surfaces of the malleoli closely approximate the sides of the trochlea in all positions from full plantar flexion to full dorsiflexion.
4. There is no appreciable lateral play of the talus within its mortise on full plantar flexion.
5. Some slight motion of the lateral malleolus (rotatory or lateral displacement or bending) can usually be perceived on dorsiflexion. The amount of this motion varies from zero to not more than 2 mm.
6. No definite relationship has yet been established between the movement of the lateral malleolus and the degree of wedging of the trochlea of the talus.
7. The curvature of the trochlea always closely approximates an arc of a circle on the lateral side and in the majority (80%) of specimens it is an arc of a circle on the medial side. The same is true of the curvature of the mortise.
8. The radius of curvature of the trochlea on its medial side is almost invariably shorter than on the lateral side. However, in spite of a shorter radius of curvature and a shorter arc on the medial side, the subtended angles are the same on the medial and lateral sides of the trochlea.
9. For all practical purposes, motion of the ankle joint can be considered to be about a single axis (this is true in 80% of the specimens, and in 20% the axis may be a changing one of not more than 10° of displacement in a transverse plane).
10. The axis of the ankle joint is obliquely oriented to the long axis of the leg.
    a. When projected on a transverse plane it is directed laterally and posteriorly.
    b. When projected on a coronal plane it is directed laterally and downward.
    c. The axis passes slightly distal to the distal tips of the malleoli.
    d. When projected upon the coronal plane, the axis bears no consistent relationship to the articular surfaces of the ankle joint.
11. The articular surfaces of the plafond and trochlea are more congruent than those of the other major articulations of the lower extremity.

5

The Conical Shape of the Trochlea

To interrelate the statements made in the preceding summary, it is necessary, as a preliminary step, to postulate a more or less plausible hypothesis. Surprisingly, such a hypothesis becomes almost self-evident when one takes an overall view of the data. The adage, "One cannot see the forest for the trees," seems particularly applicable here. The trochlea of the talus is rarely if ever a section of a cylinder, but is a section of a frustum of a cone whose apex is directed medially and whose apical angle varies considerably from individual to individual.

Support for this hypothesis can be deduced from the presently available data. The greater anteroposterior dimensions of the lateral facet and of the articular cartilage on the lateral side of the trochlea compared with the medial side are suggestive of a cone. The fact that the radius of curvature is smaller on the medial than on the lateral side of the trochlea, although the subtended angles between the radii connecting the limits of the articular cartilage are approximately the same on the two sides, can only be true in a conical structure (rather than a cylindrical one). The greater anteroposterior width of the plafond on the lateral side, as compared with the medial side, is in accord with the concept of a conical surface. Finally, Clark (1877) demonstrated that if soft wax is molded over the articular surface of the trochlea and carefully flattened, the product has the shape of a curved ribbon rather than a straight one. This could only result from molding over a conical surface rather than over a cylindrical one.

While a conical surface of the talus now appears to be more likely than a cylindrical one, a visual confirmation is afforded by rotating the talus within its mortise and making saw cuts at intervals into the trochlea as the talus is moved from full plantar flexion to full dorsiflexion. This was originally done by Close and Inman (1952), who utilized undissected cadaver ankles. These investigators demonstrated that the saw cuts were not parallel, as one would expect if the trochlea of the talus were cylindrical, but converged toward the medial side. To obtain more information, 86 cadaver ankles were studied with the use of a specially built holder and guide (Appendix E). Only those specimens showing circularity of the trochlea on both medial and lateral sides were utilized.

The converging saw cuts are readily seen in the appended photograph (Fig. 5.1) of four selected tali and the casts of their mortises. That the trochlea is a section of a frustum of a cone and not of a cylinder is clearly shown in Figures 5.2 and 5.3, in which Kirschner wires have been pressed into three of the saw cuts in each specimen. The convergence of the Kirschner wires toward the axis rod on the medial side of each talus adumbrates the cone of which each trochlea is the frustum.

The average conical angle of the saw cuts on the 86 tali was 24° ± 6° and on the cast of the mortise was 22° ± 4°. The distribution of the individual values of the apical angles is depicted in the histograms (Fig. 5.4). It should be noted that a few values of the apical angles were less than 10°. These were lumped together since the apparatus and technique used were inaccurate below this range. These specimens approximated a cylindrical shape and the apex of the cone approached infinity. Therefore, the range of the measured apical angles was considered to be from 0 to 38°.

The demonstration that the radius of curvature of the trochlea is less on the medial than on the lateral side, while the arcs of curvature of the articular surfaces, although different, subtend the same angle, together with the visual impression gained from the saw cuts and the demonstration of an angle of convergence of these saw cuts toward the medial side, seems to confirm irrefutably the basic concept that the trochlea is rarely, if ever, a section of a cylinder but rather of a frustum of a cone, whose apical angle shows considerable individual variation.

If we start from the assumption that the trochlea is conical rather than cylindrical in shape, it will be of interest to reevaluate the apparent contradictions in the literature and to reexamine certain known anatomic facts concerning the ankle.

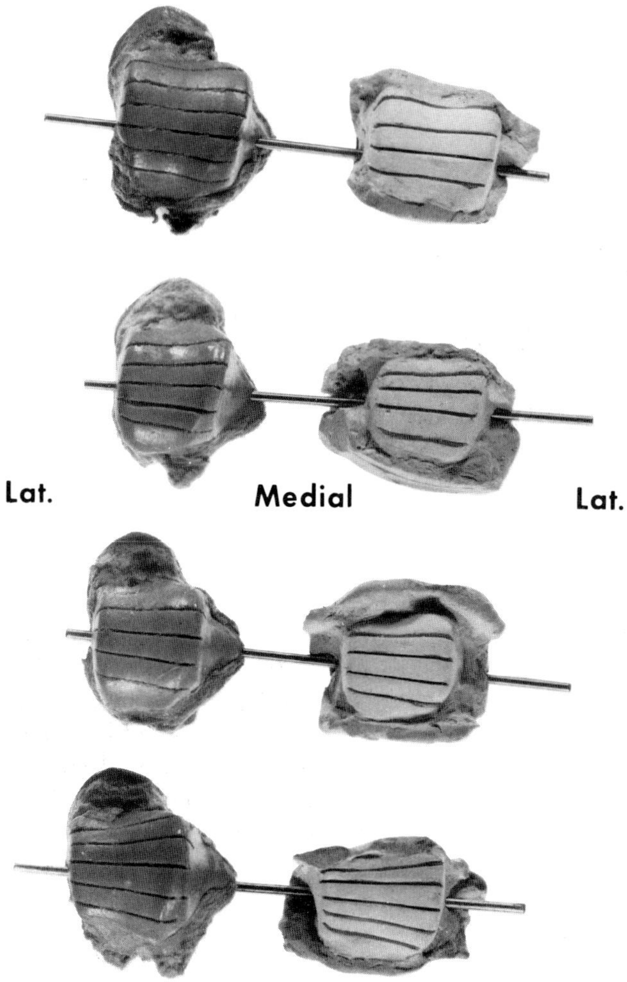

FIG. 5.1. Photographs of four selected right tali and casts of their mortises. Each talus with its cast is mounted on a single 3-mm stainless steel rod which represents the empirical axis. Note the variation in the degree of convergence of the saw cuts. In the *top photograph* the saw cuts are almost parallel, indicating that the trochlea approaches a section of a cylinder, and its cast shows that the mortise is quadrilateral in shape. The *bottom photograph* shows marked convergence of the saw cuts, and the cast shows the mortise to be trapezoidal.

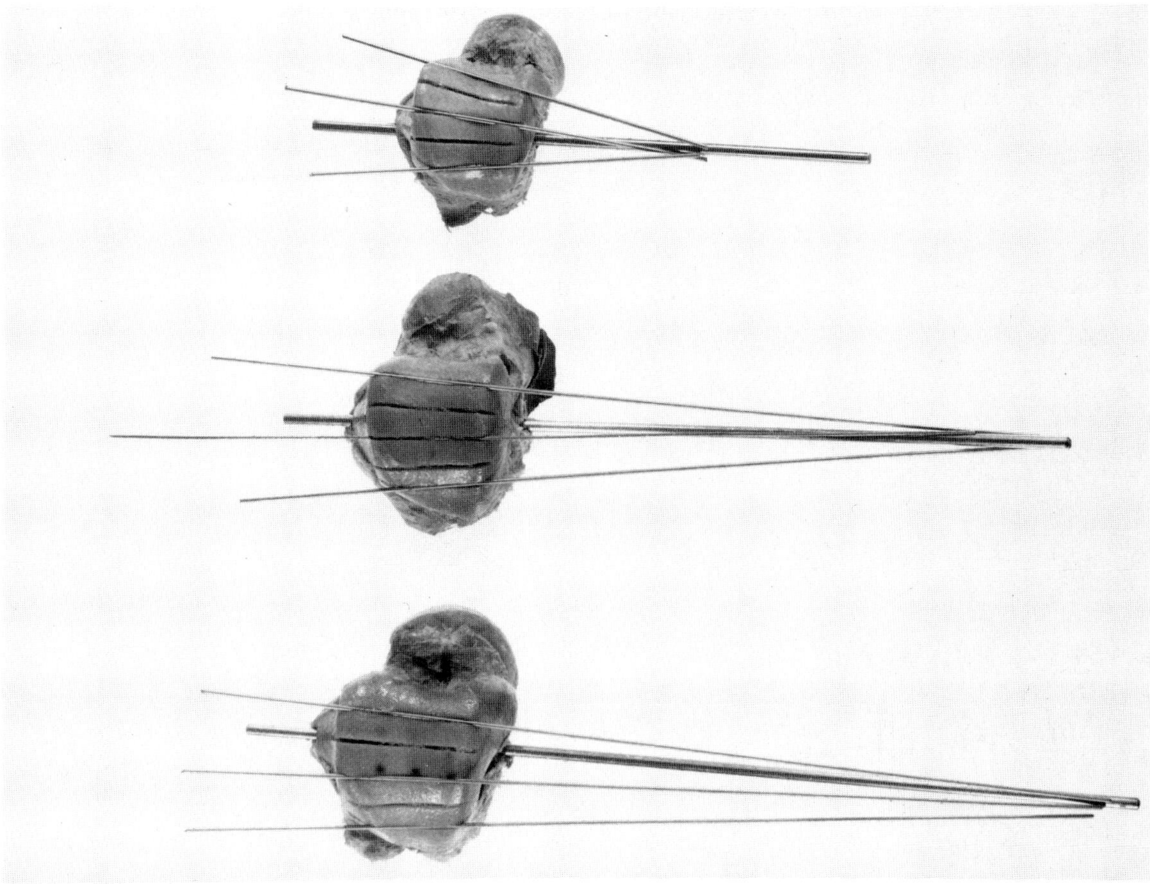

FIG. 5.2. Photographs of three selected left tali viewed from above. Kirschner wires have been pressed into the saw cuts. Note their convergence onto the stainless steel rod representing the empirical axis.

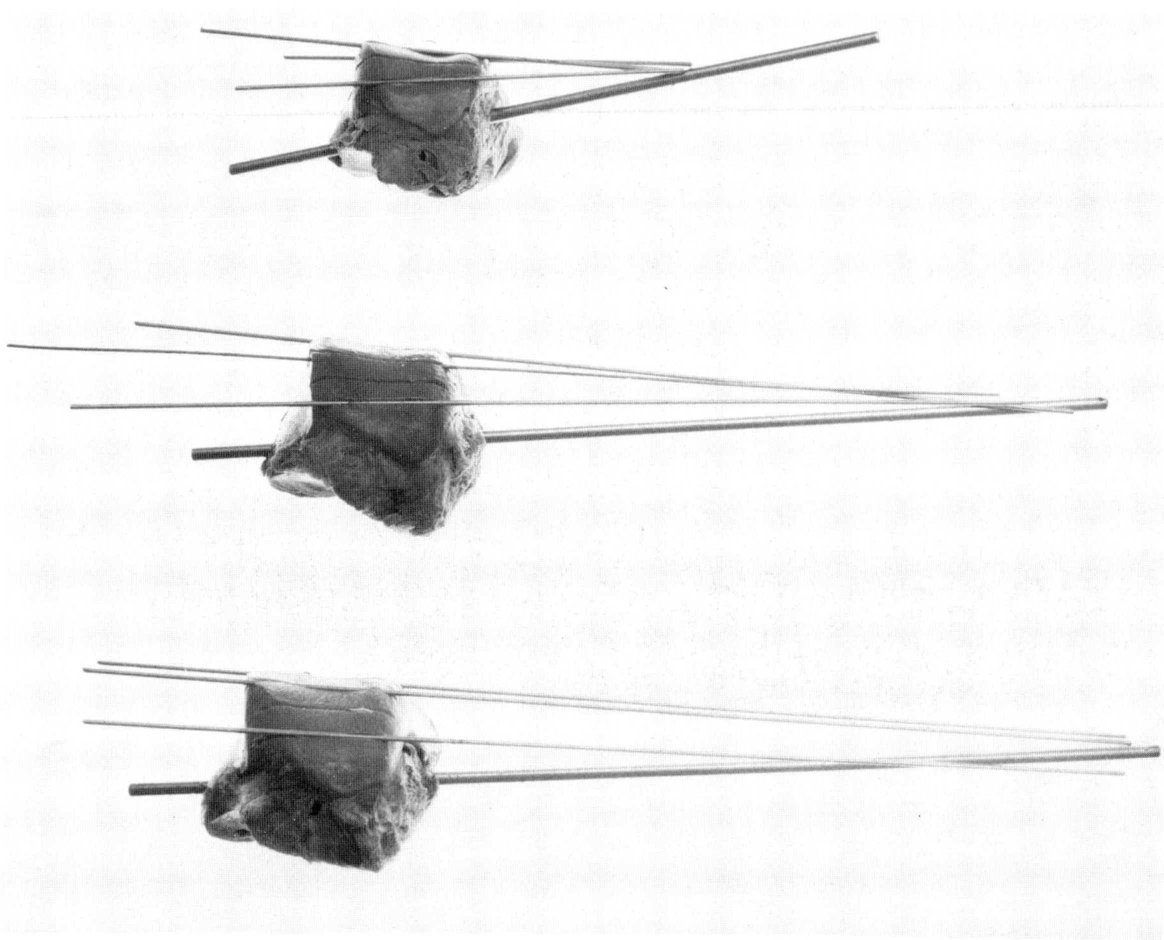

FIG. 5.3. Same specimens as in Figure 5.2, viewed from the back. Note that the Kirschner wires adumbrate half of a cone, with the rod representing the ankle axis corresponding to the axis of the cone. Note also that the obliquity of the ankle axis varies in the three tali and bears no relationship to the superior articular surface of the trochlea.

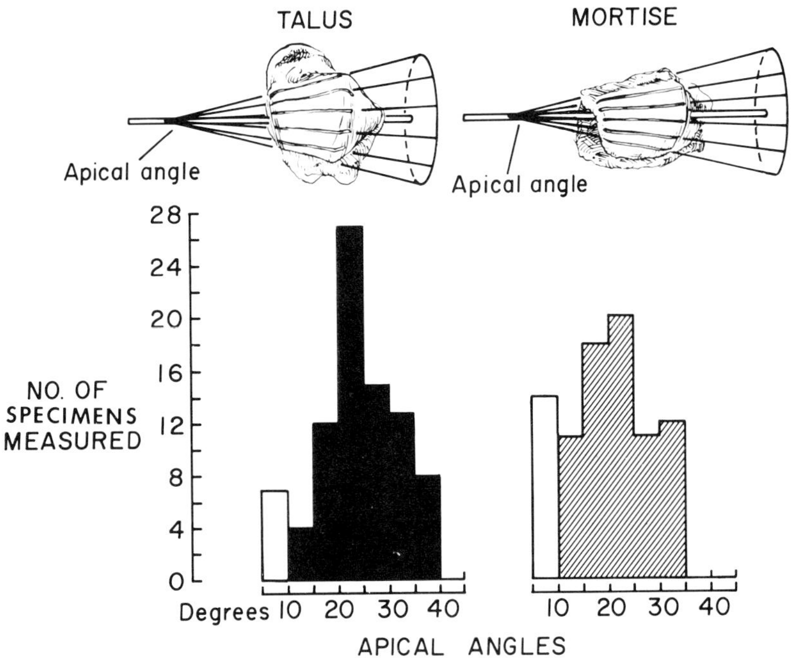

FIG. 5.4. Variations in apical angles of conical surfaces of trochleas and casts of mortises, obtained by extending directions of saw cuts toward medial sides. All specimens whose apical angles were 10° or less were lumped together and are shown in the *clear bars* of the *histograms*.

6

Reassessment of the Question of Malleolar Separation and the Wedge Shape of the Trochlea

All previous investigators appear to have measured the transverse width of the trochlea in planes perpendicular to the tibial facet. For the study of the isolated talus this seemed to be the most natural procedure, since the tibial articular facet appears to parallel the long axis of the bone and presents a flatter surface than that of the fibular facet, which could therefore be employed as a reference plane. However, the angle between the plane of the tibial facet and the functional axis of the ankle has been shown to vary considerably from specimen to specimen. Different orientations in the measured widths in relation to the functional axis of the ankle could be a source of discrepancies. Therefore, it appears more reasonable to measure the widths, with the saw cuts in the trochlea as directional guides; these at least would orient the measurements along the conical surface of the trochlea.

This was done (Appendix E), and the gross variation in the widths of the trochlea reported in previous studies miraculously seemed to disappear. In all specimens the differences in the widths from the most anterior to the most posterior saw cut were reduced to zero or at least were halved (*i.e.*, they were less than 2 mm). If the most anterior saw cut was compared with the center cut, the difference in measurement in any one specimen was negligible (within the limits of accuracy of measurement, or $\pm$ 1 mm). The same results were obtained when the middle saw cut was compared with the most posterior cut.

It should be remembered that during full flexion and extension of the ankle, the mortise is only required to accept slightly over half of the trochlea at any one time. Since the true functional widths of the trochlea are smaller than previously assumed, it is easy to see how a very small motion of the lateral malleolus is all that is required during movement of the talus in its mortise. The actual recorded motion of the lateral malleolus (less than 2 mm) (Ashhurst and Bromer, 1922; Close and Inman, 1952; Close, 1956; Grath, 1960) is all that is necessary to accommodate the most extremely wedge-shaped talus. The lateral movement of the fibular malleolus or its rotation about a vertical axis or the slight bending of the fibula, which have all been reported to occur, need be only barely perceptible. The changes in the mortise require at most a millimeter to adjust to the trochlea since the reported disparities in widths of the trochlea are in reality nonexistent. Also it is understandable that Barnett and Napier (1952) failed to find any relationship between movement of the fibular malleolus and the degree of wedging of the trochlea. The various theoretical explanations proposed in the literature and expounded in some textbooks to account for the assumed disparity in the widths of the trochlea are not, in fact, necessary.

In addition, one is not surprised that rigid fixation of a diastasis of the distal tibiofibular syndesmosis by bolts, screws, or bone grafts has in most cases resulted in little disability. Single examples of screws breaking, loosening, or eroding into the cortex of the fibula are depicted in several textbooks when fractures about the ankle are discussed. This is understandable since some fibulas do move slightly, but the intriguing fact is that rigid internal fixation results in no disability in the vast majority of persons treated in this manner for diastasis of the tibiofibular syndesmosis. If a fear that restricted motion in the ankle will result from rigid internal fixation still persists in the mind of the surgeon, this fear can be somewhat alleviated by fully dorsiflexing the ankle at the time the bolt, screw, or wire is finally tightened.

Furthermore, the widely published assertions, in clinical texts, that there is increased lateral play of the talus in plantar flexion, and the failure of investigators who have specifically studied this possibility to support such a statement, are a remarkable journalistic phenomenon. One can not suppress the feeling that some authors have been guilty of whimsical and capricious thinking. The concept of the trochlea being a section of a frustum of a cone obviates the need to postulate an increase in lateral movement of the talus when the foot is plantar flexed and explains the constant contact of the malleolar facets with the sides of the trochlea during the entire range of motion of the ankle.

7

Obliquity of the Ankle Axis in Relation to the Long Axis of the Tibia

When an isolated tibia is inspected or an anteroposterior roentgenogram of the ankle is examined, it appears that the articular surface of the tibia lies in a plane that is at nearly a right angle to the long axis of the bone. Isman and Inman (1968) measured the angle between the midline of the tibia and the plane of the plafond of the tibia. Their method was indirect and its accuracy was questionable. Their series was reinvestigated and additional specimens were measured with a more direct method (see Appendix A). In 107 cadaver specimens the angle measured in the coronal plane on the medial side between the midline of the tibia and the surface of the plafond of the ankle was found to be 93.3° ± 3.2°, with a range of 88 to 100° (Fig. 7.1).

The angle between the empirical axis of the ankle joint (Appendix A) and the midline of the tibia in the same series of specimens was 82.7° ± 3.7°, with a range of 74 to 94° (Fig. 7.2).

The average angular difference between the empiri-

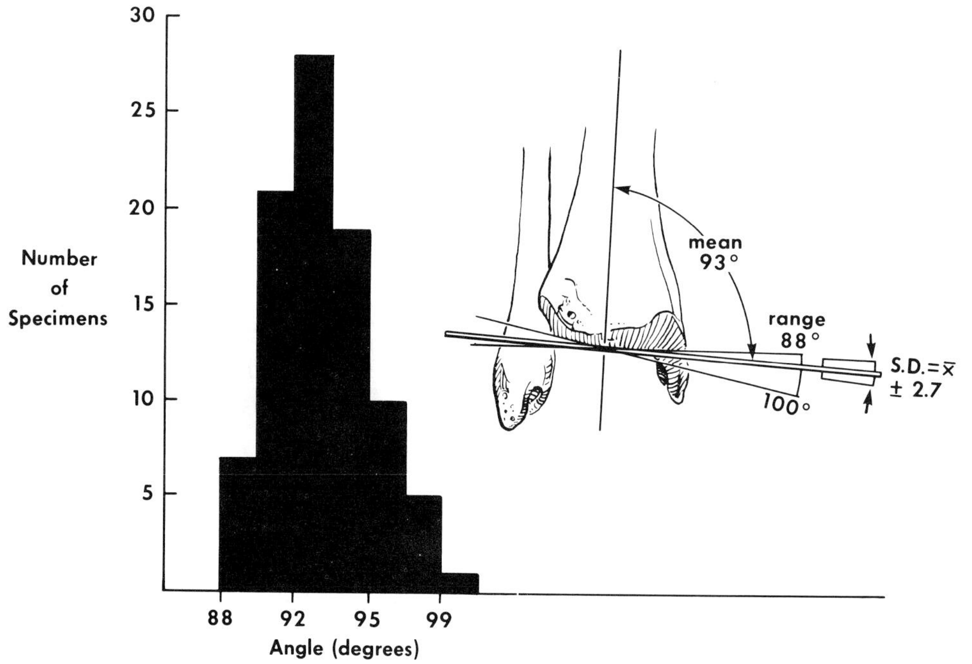

FIG. 7.1. Variations in angle between midline of tibia and plafond of mortise. The distribution of the values is shown in the *histogram*. Note the small amount of spread among the individual measurements (approximately 10°).

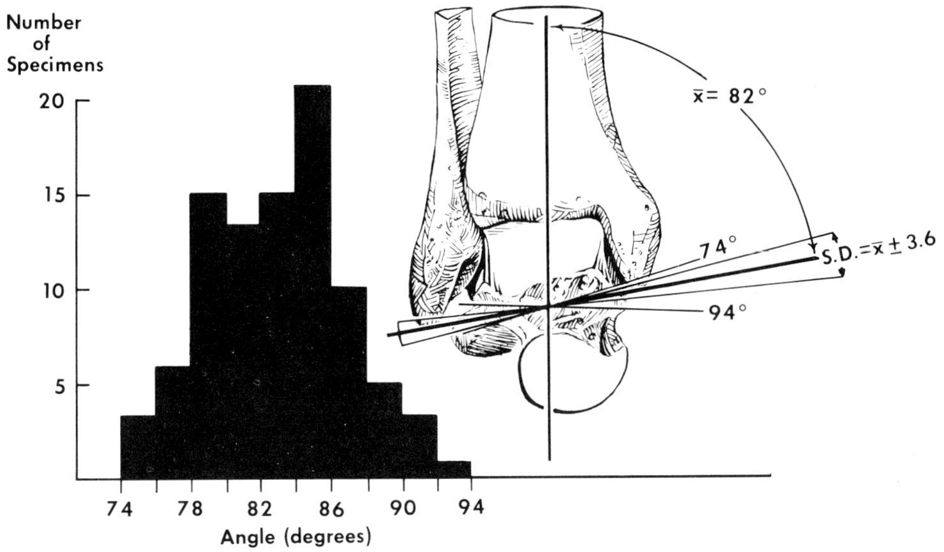

FIG. 7.2. Variations in angle between midline of tibia and empirical axis of ankle. The *histogram* reveals a considerable spread of individual values.

cal axis and the plane of the plafond of the tibia was found to be 11.3° ± 4.1°, with a range of 2 to 21°. This means that in all the specimens the empirical axis was oblique to the articular surface of the ankle joint. This agrees with and confirms the findings of Barnett and Napier (1952). While these investigators did not state in the text of their publication the precise relationship of the axis to the malleoli, they clearly depict it in one of their sketches as passing, when projected on the coronal plane, just distal to the tips of both malleoli. In our series the empirical axis was also found to pass slightly distal to the tips of the malleoli. However, the relationship of the empirical axis to the malleolar tips was not absolutely invariable. On the medial side the axis passed, on the average, 5 ± 3 mm (range, 0 to 11 mm) distal to the distal tip of the medial malleolus; on the lateral side, the axis passed 3 ± 2 mm (range, 0 to 12 mm) distal to and 8 ± 5 mm anterior to the distal tip of the lateral malleolus. While these measurements reveal considerable individual variation, one can categorically state that the axis of the ankle is oblique in the coronal plane and passes slightly distal to each malleolus. For clinical purposes one can press a finger under the tip of each malleolus (Fig. 7.3) or on an anteroposterior x-ray connect the distal ends of the two malleoli (Fig. 7.4) and determine with reasonable accuracy the inclination of the ankle axis as projected on the coronal plane.

Dunn and Samuelson (1974), in their study of the flat-top talus, provided additional evidence to support the contention that the axis of the ankle passes close to the tips of the malleoli. In 14 normal patients the foot was rotated medially at 10° intervals. The

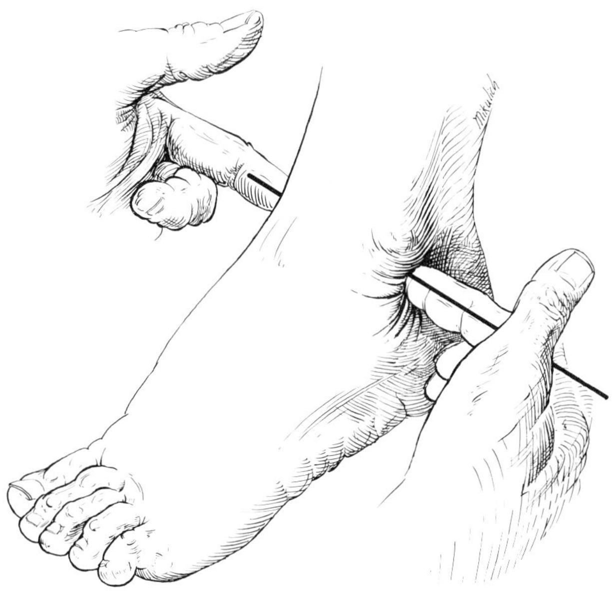

FIG. 7.3. Estimation of position of ankle axis by palpation of malleoli. (Reproduced with permission, from Inman, Verne T., and Mann, Roger A. Biomechanics of the foot and ankle. In Inman, Verne T. (ed.) *DuVries' Surgery of the Foot*. Ed. 3, The C.V. Mosby Company, St. Louis, 1973)

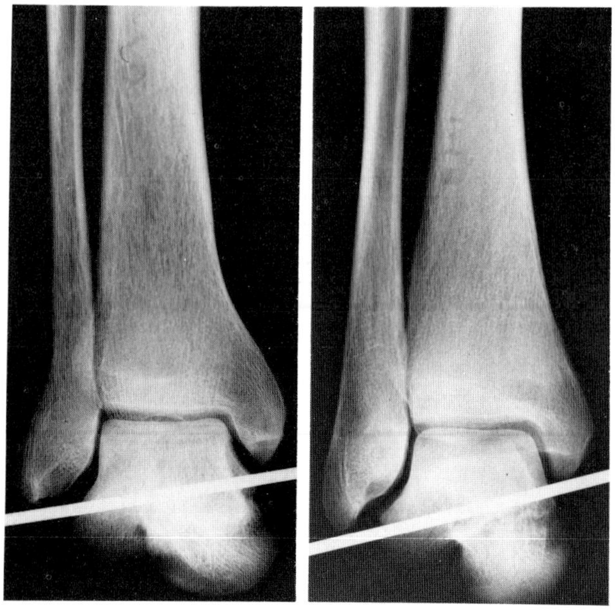

FIG. 7.4. Anteroposterior x-rays of two randomly selected cadaver ankles. It can be clearly seen that the rod representing the empirically determined ankle axis passes just below the tips of the two malleoli.

authors reported that "the true lateral anatomy of the talus could best be demonstrated with the foot medially rotated sufficiently to superimpose the medial and lateral malleoli." In so doing these investigators were inadvertently lining up the axis of the ankle to lie vertically to the plane of the film.

When it is appreciated that the trochlea is a section of a frustum rather than of a cylinder, one can readily appreciate that the obliquity of the axis can vary from individual to individual even though the articular surfaces of the ankle joint appear to lie in a plane perpendicular to the long axis of the leg (see Fig. 5.3).

8

Explanations for Certain Anatomic Features

The concept that the trochlea is in reality a section of a frustum of a cone rather than of a cylinder appears to provide at least a partial explanation for certain anatomic features exhibited by both skeletal and ligamentous structures in and about the ankle joint. These would be difficult to understand if the trochlea were a cylinder.

As stated above, the anteroposterior lengths of the articular facets on the two sides of the trochlea differ. The tibial facet is usually small, short, and comma-shaped, and often terminates short of the posterior limits of the articular cartilage on the superior surface of the trochlea. The fibular facet is longer and always extends the entire length of the articular surface. This is exactly the situation one would expect to find if the trochlea were a section of a frustum, since the medial malleolus lies closer to the apex of the cone and for the same angular motion of the ankle would have less anteroposterior displacement than the base of the lateral malleolus, which lies farther from the apex.

When the superior surface of the talus is observed, the length of the arc of the trochlea appears to be greater on the lateral than on the medial side, and measurement has shown this to be true. Again, this is what one would expect on viewing a conical surface; the lengths of the arcs would increase with increasing distance from the apex of the cone. The mortise reveals similar differences. Casts of the mortises disclose their trapezoidal shapes, with the lateral side being longer than the medial side. Photographs of 10 randomly selected casts are shown in Figure 8.1. The differences in the anteroposterior dimensions on the medial and lateral sides are apparent and indicate that the reciprocal surface of the plafond must also be conical.

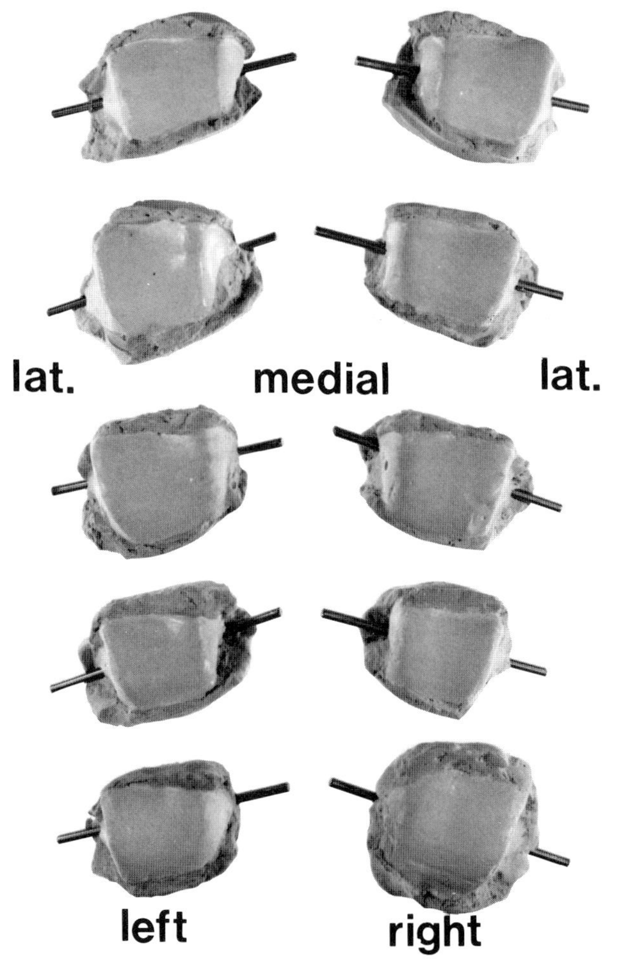

FIG. 8.1. Photographs of 10 randomly selected casts of mortises of ankle joints. Note their trapezoidal shape. The anteroposterior dimensions are greater on the lateral than on the medial sides, suggesting conical surfaces.

Furthermore, when the talus is viewed from above, the tibial facet on the medial side of the trochlea usually appears to be relatively straight and to lie in a flat vertical plane. The fibular facet on the lateral side, however, appears to curve (Fig. 8.2). This configuration gives the trochlea its wedge-shaped appearance. The explanation for these differences in the two facets seems to be simply a matter of projection. An attempt is made to visually demonstrate this by inserting a talus inside of a transparent glass cone. The sides of the glass cone parallel the Kirschner wires which denote the conical shape of the enclosed talus. The glass cone, by being a complete cone and larger in size, more clearly demonstrates the necessity for a curvilinear shape to the fibular facet. Reference to Figure 8.3 should make clear this otherwise obscure relationship.

A pictorial review appears appropriate at this time to summarize what appears to be the proper concept of the structure of the trochlea of the talus. This is shown in Figure 8.4.

The lateral malleolus extends farther distally than does the medial malleolus. The reason for this anatomic fact is difficult to understand if the axis of the ankle joint is assumed to lie in a transverse plane and perpendicular to the leg. An oblique axis, however, makes such an anatomic arrangement almost obligatory. The skeletal attachments of the collateral ligaments should lie close to the axis of motion where they would be subjected to minimal spatial displacement. An oblique axis and a minimal displacement of the ligaments can only obtain if the malleoli are of different lengths.

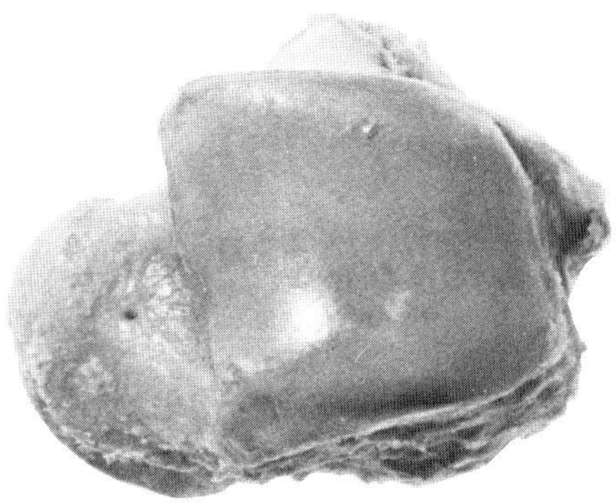

FIG. 8.2. Top view of a typical talus. The superior surface of the trochlea has been oriented to lie in a horizontal plane and perpendicular to the line of sight of the camera. Note that the edges between the superior surface of the trochlea and the two malleolar facets differ on the two sides. On the tibial side the edge appears to be relatively straight while on the fibular side the edge is gently curved, giving a wedge-shaped appearance to the superior surface of the trochlea.

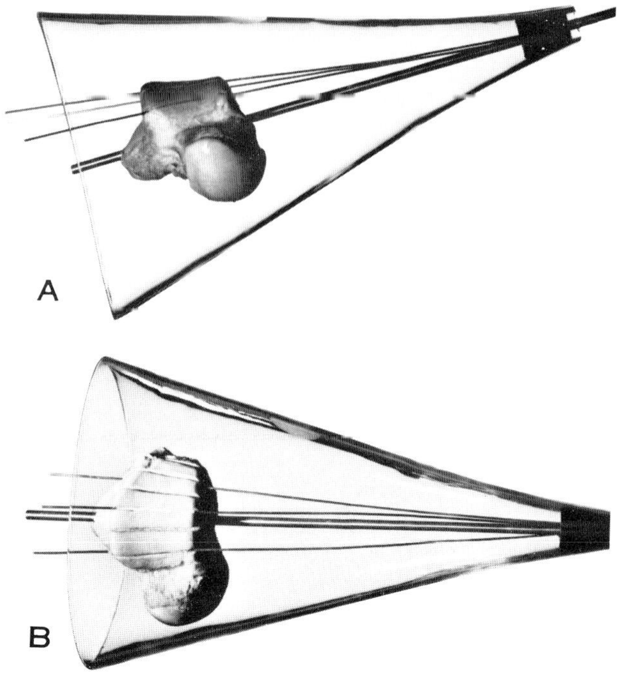

FIG. 8.3. *A*, Talus mounted inside transparent glass cone and oriented so it is viewed from front. Note that while the superior surface of the trochlea is horizontal, the axis is oblique, causing both the glass cone and the conical surface of the trochlea, as adumbrated by the Kirschner wires, to be slanted. *B*, View from above of glass cone with enclosed talus, which has not been moved. Note that because of the obliquity of the axis and the slant of the glass cone (*A*), the open base of the glass cone is now viewed as an ellipse. Attention is called to the resultant parallelism between the edge of the glass cone and the curvature of the lateral edge of the trochlea.

When teaching anatomy, the author was always puzzled by the differences in the distal projections of the two malleoli. The concept of a transverse axis paralleling the joint surface led to difficulties in understanding the function of the collateral ligaments. If the axis passed through the lateral malleolus above the attachment of the lateral collateral ligaments, then the tip of the malleolus would be displaced forward and backward with ankle motion and the ligaments would be subjected to alternating tensions and relaxations. This could never be satisfactorily demonstrated in the cadaver. A similar situation for the deltoid ligament would exist if the axis passed too far distal to the medial malleolus. However, an oblique axis which passes close to the attachments of both medial and lateral collateral ligaments to their respective malleoli obviates this difficulty.

Finally, a further observation may explain some of the differences in the construction of the tibial and

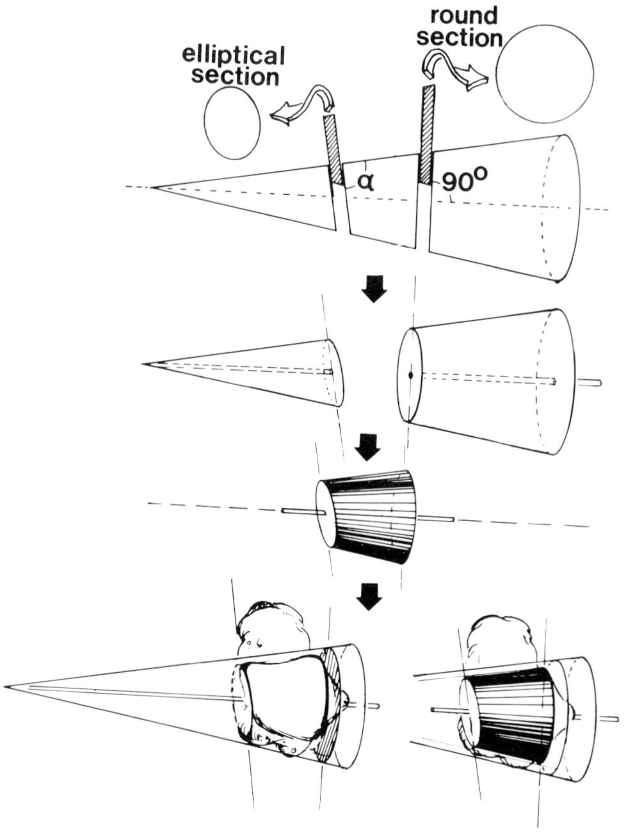

FIG. 8.4. Pictorial representation of present concept of construction of trochlea of talus. A frustum is cut from a cone. The section cut at 90° to the axis of the cone is circular when projected onto a transverse plane of the cone (see Barnett and Napier, 1952); this corresponds to the fibular (lateral) facet. The section cut obliquely is elliptical; this corresponds to the tibial (medial) facet. Note that the fibular facet, being farther from the apex of the cone, possesses greater dimensions. With minor modifications, a section of the frustum is converted into the trochlea of the talus. The anteroposterior curve of the fibular facet is an ellipse because of the oblique orientation of the conical surface of the trochlea when viewed from above.

the fibular collateral ligaments. The medial malleolus, being closer to the apex of the cone of which the trochlea is a frustum, exhibits less anteroposterior excursion, and the fibers constituting the collateral ligament can be concentrated into a single deltoid structure. While conceivably a similar mechanical arrangement could exist on the lateral side, such is not the case. The lateral collateral ligament is composed of three distinct and separate structures: the anterior and posterior talofibular and the calcaneofibular ligaments. The reason for such an anatomic arrangement is not readily apparent. The fibular attachments of these three ligaments are in line with the oblique axis of the ankle joint which passes close beneath the tip of the lateral malleolus. Therefore the normal flexion and extension movements of the ankle lead to little or no changes in tension of these structures. Why then should there exist three independent ligaments which arise from the malleolus close to the ankle axis but diverge widely at their more distal skeletal attachments? It appears reasonable to surmise that certain evolutionary factors were involved in the development of the present arrangement in man. A search of the literature, however, was disappointing. Comparative anatomic studies which describe the ligaments of the ankle in other primates are infrequent and sketchy. This was noted by Keith (1893–1894), who stated, "Notwithstanding the very considerable amount which has been written concerning the bones, muscles, and brain, . . . ligaments have been mentioned in only an incidental manner. It is not that the ligaments merit this neglect, for perhaps of all structures they are the most susceptible of adaptative influences, and even in a rudimentary condition they are most persistent." With this thought in mind, it would perhaps be of interest to explore separately, as far as is possible with our present knowledge, the comparative anatomy of the three fascicles which together comprise the lateral collateral ligament of the ankle joint.

In old world monkeys (Cynomorpha) Keith reported that all three divisions of the fibular collateral ligaments were present but the anterior talofibular ligament was weak. Hill (1960) found that in primates the posterior (posterior talofibular) and the middle (calcaneofibular) fasciculi were well marked, but that the anterior (anterior talofibular) fascicle was only feebly represented or was lacking. A dissection made by us of an ankle of a Macaque revealed well-developed calcaneofibular and posterior talofibular ligaments (Fig. 8.5*A* and *B*) but not even a suggestion of an anterior talofibular ligament (Fig. 8.5*C*). The chimpanzee, whose general skeletal structure most closely resembles man's, still retains an essentially quadrupedal type of locomotion. Jones (1929) states that these animals "shuffle along on flexed legs with the knuckles of the manus completing the quadrupedal poise which is habitual." A dissection of the lateral ligaments of the ankle reveals well-developed posterior talofibular and calcaneofibular ligaments but no evidence of an anterior talofibular ligament (Fig. 8.6).

Hill ventures to state that the anterior talofibular ligament "differentiated in adaptation to the orthograde posture." Should the development of an anterior talofibular ligament be related to a plantigrade type of locomotion it becomes of interest to investigate the anatomy of the lateral ligaments in those animals which most closely approximate man in this kind of locomotion. The gibbon, normally an arboreal acrobat, with his relatively long arms, when walking or running on the ground has a remarkably humanoid

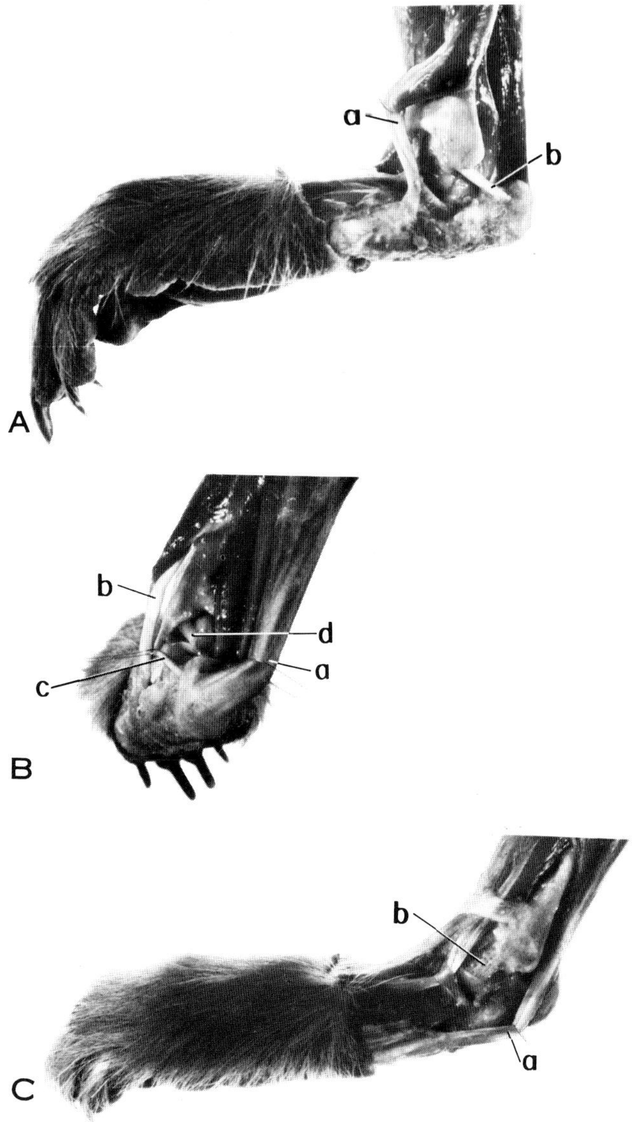

FIG. 8.5. Dissection of ankle of rhesus macaque (*Macaca mulatta*). *A*, Peroneal tendons retracted forward out of their groove behind lateral malleolus (*a*). A well-developed calcaneofibular ligament (*b*) can be distinctly seen passing from the tip of the lateral malleolus obliquely backward and downward to the calcaneus. *B*, Calcaneal tendon (*a*) retracted medially. The peroneal tendons (*b*) have been displaced anterolaterally and the calcaneofibular ligament (*c*) has been retracted. The posterior talofibular ligament (*d*) is now visible, extending from the deep surface of the lateral malleolus to the posterior surface of the talus. *C*, Anterolateral view of same specimen. The thin anterior capsule of the ankle joint was removed in the dissection during the search for any evidence of an anterior talofibular ligament; none was found. The peroneal tendons (*a*) have been retracted to expose the head and neck of the talus (*b*).

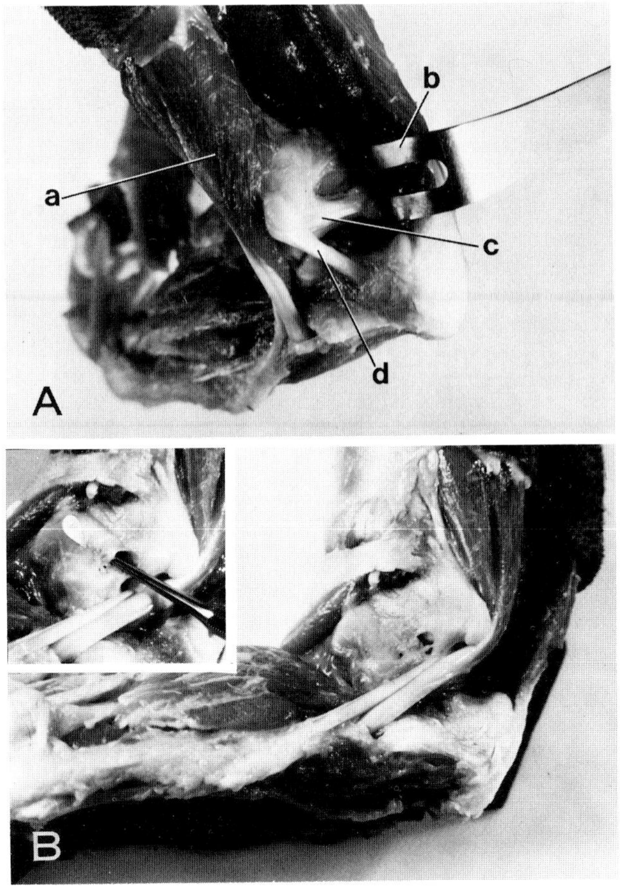

FIG. 8.6. Dissection of ankle of chimpanzee. *A*, Posterolateral view. The peroneal muscles and tendons (*a*) have been displaced anteriorly from their groove in the posterior surface of the lateral malleolus. The triceps surae muscle and the calcaneal tendon (*b*) have been retracted medially to expose the posterior aspect of the ankle. A well-developed posterior talofibular ligament (*c*) and calcaneofibular ligament (*d*) are clearly seen. *B*, Anterolateral view. Note, anteriorly, the thin anterior capsule of the ankle joint, through which the anterior portion of the trochlea can be seen. The *inset* shows a small surgical elevator inserted under the lateral portion of the capsule, revealing some slight thickening but no definite anterior talofibular ligament.

gait. While holding his long arms abducted from his upright body, he appears to be truly plantigrade. Dissections of the ankle reveal all three fascicles of the lateral ligament to be present in an arrangement that is surprisingly human (Fig 8.7). The bear, whose hindfoot resembles man's in several ways, having a longitudinal arch and being definitely plantigrade, reveals not only the presence of a posterior talofibular and a distinct calcaneofibular ligament (Fig. 8.8*A*), but also a definite thickening in the anterior capsule of the ankle which resembles the anterior talofibular ligament in man, except that in this specimen it is bifid (Fig. 8.8*B*). There is also an accessory peroneal muscle whose tendon passes anterior to the malleolus

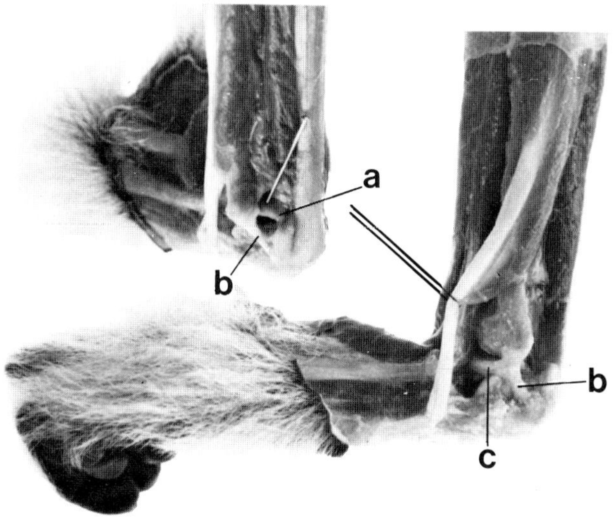

FIG. 8.7. Dissection of ankle of gibbon (*Hylobates lar*). The *inset* is a posterolateral view and shows the posterior talofibular ligament (*a*), in which a pin has been inserted, and the calcaneofibular ligament (*b*). The anterolateral view reveals a strong anterior talofibular ligament (*c*).

and which tends to parallel the fibers of the anterior talofibular ligament with full plantar flexion of the ankle. By its contraction it could restrict inversion of the foot and prevent overstretching of the anterior talofibular ligament when the foot is plantar flexed. If it is true that the appearance of a powerful anterior talofibular ligament in man is the consequence of his bipedal plantigrade type of locomotion then two inferences appear possible. The anterior talofibular ligament must play a particularly significant role in the stabilization of the human ankle, but precisely how it functions is subject to conjecture at this time. However, it is interesting that it is the first to suffer injury from inversion sprains of the ankle (Leonard, 1949), which further suggests that it functions in some particular manner to restrict medial tilting of the talus in its mortise.

Little information relative to the posterior talofibular ligament is obtained from a review of the literature. Comparative anatomic studies are lacking. When mentioned at all, a simple statement is made that this ligament is present as a distinct structure in all primate and prosimian species. Its precise function in the stabilization of the talus is based purely on conjecture, and injury to this ligament is relatively uncommon (Ashhurst and Bromer, 1922; Anderson and LeCocq, 1954; Francillon, 1962; Bonnin, 1965).

The calcaneofibular ligament is a particularly interesting structure; its anatomic arrangement and its involvement in both ankle and subtalar function warrant a detailed discussion. This ligament is present as a distinct and separate structure in all primate

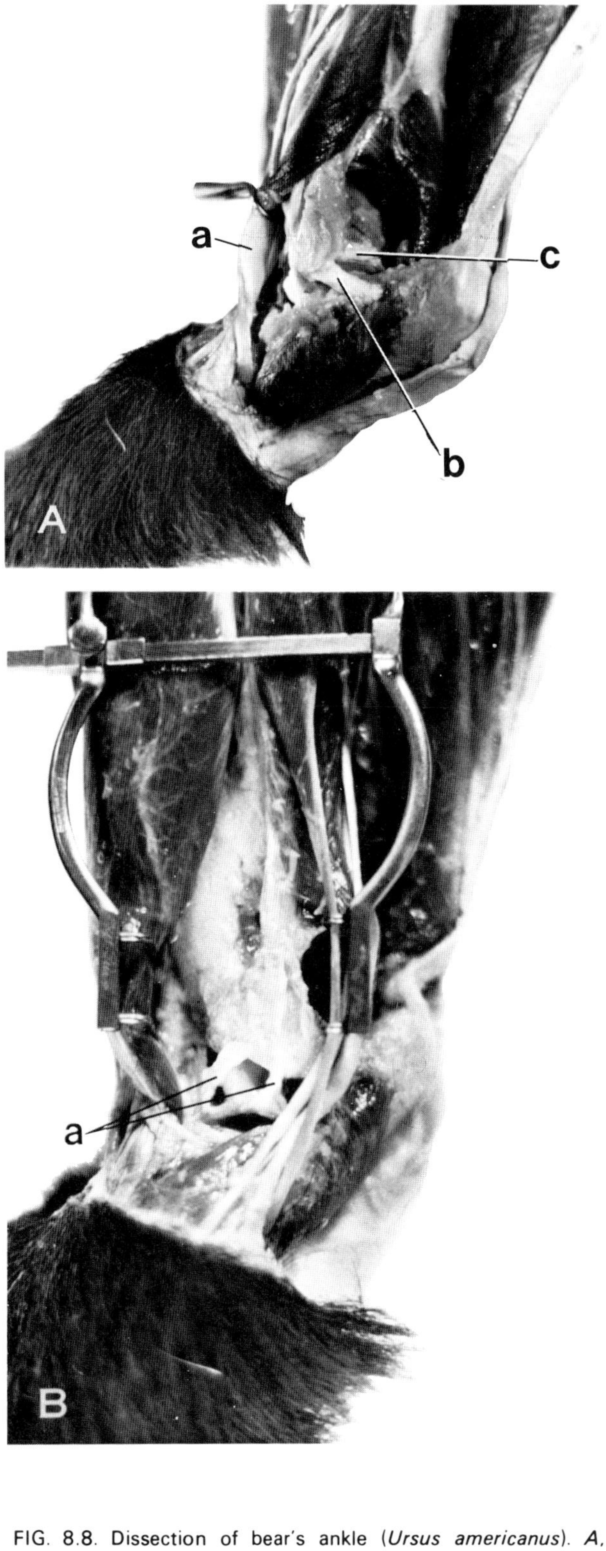

FIG. 8.8. Dissection of bear's ankle (*Ursus americanus*). *A*, Lateral view. The peroneal tendons (*a*) have been retracted, revealing the presence of a calcaneofibular ligament (*b*) and a posterior talofibular ligament (*c*). *B*, Anterolateral view. The dissection revealed two definite thickenings (*a*) in the capsule of the ankle joint, which extended from the anterior surface of the lateral malleolus to the articular edge of the trochlea of the talus.

and prosimian species. Therefore it "can boast a noble descent" (Bland-Sutton, 1897).

In sections dealing with syndesmology, all texts and atlases classify the calcaneofibular ligament as belonging exclusively to the ankle joint and invariably depict it with the ankle in the anatomic position, *i.e.*, with the foot at a right angle to the leg. This is a too simplistic presentation and fails to convey an adequate understanding of the contribution of this structure to the function and stability of the ankle joint. It is most important to remember that the calcaneofibular ligament passes over two joints and is as much related to the subtalar as to the ankle joint. Only when this fact is appreciated does the anatomic disposition of this ligament and its changing contribution to the stability of the ankle become clear.

The illustrations in the standard textbooks of anatomy (*e.g.*, Quain, 1867; Cunningham, 1964; Morris, 1966; Gray, 1973) and the time-honored atlases (*e.g.*, Toldt, 1914; Sobotta, 1957) show the calcaneofibular ligament passing from its fibular attachment downward and backward to the calcaneus. In many of the simpler texts, where pen-and-ink sketches are used, the calcaneofibular ligament is depicted as a true collateral ligament passing from the lateral malleolus directly downward to the calcaneus; this representation is anatomically untrue and functionally impossible. Only Fick (1904) emphasized the oblique course of this ligament, stating, "*Nie habe ich das Band vertikal laufen sehen, . . . sondern meist macht es nach meinen Messungen mit der Horizontalen einen Winkel von weniger als 45°.*"

Both skeletal attachments of this ligament are critical. The empirical axis of the ankle joint has been demonstrated to pass close to the tip of the fibular malleolus (Isman and Inman, 1968; see also Appendix A). Flexion and extension of the ankle about this axis cause little or no displacement of the tip of the malleolus relative to the remainder of the foot. The calcaneofibular ligament, being attached to the tip of the malleolus and hence close to the axis of motion, is subjected to no undue tensions during the full ranges of motion of the ankle joint. The necessity for the calcaneofibular ligament to pursue an oblique course, backward and downward, to its calcaneal attachment is at first glance not readily apparent. Only when it is realized that its direction is dictated by subtalar motion and not ankle motion does its anatomic arrangement become understandable.

Therefore, further consideration concerning the anatomic disposition and the functional significance of the calcaneofibular ligament must be deferred until certain facts pertaining to the subtalar joint are presented. This is done in the next chapter. The discussion on the calcaneofibular ligament will be presented later (pages 70–73).

9

The Subtalar Joint

Before proceeding with a discussion of the subtalar joint, it should be emphasized that the talus plays a unique role in the functional anatomy of the lower extremity; it is the link between the leg and the foot. The ankle joint constitutes its proximal connection to the leg and the subtalar joint is its distal connection to the foot. It is appreciated that the movement of the talus produces, in addition, important and definitive effects upon the foot through its distal articulation with the navicular. However, there was never any intention to expand this monograph to include a discussion of the functional anatomy of the foot, and the effect of movement of the talus upon the transverse tarsal articulations (the talonavicular and the calcaneocuboid joints), which are so important in the function of the foot, will not be discussed.

MOTION AT THE SUBTALAR JOINT

Considerable confusion seems to persist, particularly in the English and American texts, as to the type of movement that occurs between the talus and the calcaneus—at least, the statements in most of the standard textbooks of anatomy are vague and often ambiguous. This failure to enunciate a clear description of the type of motion between these two bones appears to be due to several factors. In some cases there seems to be an outright lack of knowledge of the true nature of the motion, or the motion is described in such imprecise language that a clear understanding is not conveyed. There is also the tendency to describe the movement in terms referable to the planes of space that are external to the body, which necessarily complicates the description.

While it is not intended to burden the reader with extensive documentation, it seems appropriate to review in a cursory manner the types of statement found in textbooks of anatomy. Frazer (1933) states that the disposition of the articular surfaces "hinders any rocking or lateral movement of the bones" but that the "astragalus can be moved forwards and inwards on the os calcis." The implication appears to be that no rotation is possible—only the sliding forward and backward of the talus upon the calcaneus. A similar statement is found in Gray's *Anatomy of the Human Body* (in the 1st as well as in the 29th edition); the latter says: "The movements permitted between the talus and calcaneus are limited to gliding of the one bone on the other anteroposteriorly and from side to side" (Gray, 1973). Some texts imply that some type of rotation occurs between the talus and the calcaneus but are not too specific about the precise location of an axis. Cunningham (1927) states, "There is rotation between the talus and calcaneus about an oblique axis which passes from the medial side of the neck of the talus to the lateral and inferior part of the calcaneus." Piersol (1923) indicates the motion between the talus and calcaneus in the following quotation: "They [the motions of the subastragaloid joints] are resolved into turning on an oblique axis running through the interosseous ligament, somewhat internal to its middle, downward with something of a backward and inward inclination." Quain (1892) is more specific: "The movement between the astragalus and calcaneum is a rotation about an axis which is directed obliquely from the upper and inner part of the neck of the astragalus, backwards, downwards, and outwards, to the lower and outer part of the tuberosity of the os calcis." Cunningham (1964) states that the "axis of movement . . . runs obliquely forwards, upwards, and medially through the sinus tarsi, in the region of the ligamentum cervicis." *Grant's Method of Anatomy* (1971) quotes Hicks (1953) and depicts the axis in a line sketch of the talus and calcaneus. Hollinshead (1967) simply states, "The subtalar joint is particularly important because . . . it allows inversion and eversion of the posterior part of the foot."

The German textbooks of anatomy, while revealing some variations, are in general more specific in their descriptions. Rauber-Kopsch (1968) presents a sketch with a line indicating an axis of rotation entitled "*Bewegungen im unteren Sprunggelenk*" but with no discussion in the text. On the other hand, an earlier edition (Rauber, 1906) is quite specific in its description of an axis of rotation. Besides a drawing of the skeleton of the foot with a single axis clearly indicated, he makes the statement that the axis "*ist ungefähr 45° zum Horizont geneigt.*"

Braus (1954) also refers to a sketch indicating the axis about which the talus moves on the calcaneus and states that the range of motion averages 13°. Benninghoff and Goerttler (1960) clearly depict a single oblique axis in two line drawings and state that the compromise axis, "*die vorn medial in den Sprungbeinhals eintritt, den Sinus tarsi kreuzt und an der lateralen Seite des Fersenbeinhöckers wieder herauskommt.*"

Of the German texts, that by von Lanz and Wachsmuth (1938) is the most specific in its discussion of the subtalar joint. Relying on the published works of previous German investigators, these authors pictorially and by description state that the movement between the talus and the calcaneus is a rotation about a single oblique axis that passes through the neck of the talus, crosses the sinus tarsi, and emerges on the lateral aspect of the calcaneus. They further state that the only motion possible is rotation of the bones about this axis.

The French and Italian textbooks of anatomy discuss the movement between the talus and the calcaneus in a manner similar to the German. Charpy *et al.* (1899) depict the rotation between the two bones in a sketch and state, "*Ces mouvements s'exécutent autour d'un axe antéro-postérieur; leur centre répond à l'insertion du ligament interosseux dans la gouttière calcanéenne.*" Paturet (1951) includes a sketch that shows the axis as projected onto a transverse plane and gives a short discussion of the rotation. Rouvière (1962) quotes Charpy *et al.* (cited by him as Poirier). Bairati (1963) quotes von Lanz and Wachsmuth and reproduces one of the drawings from their atlas.

Inspection of the talus with its "bewildering congeries of articular surfaces" (Elftman and Manter, 1935) has made it difficult to visualize the motion between the talus and calcaneus. But these authors should be given credit for introducing to the English literature the concepts of the position of the subtalar axis and the true type of motion between the talus and the calcaneus. And every investigator who has carefully studied the motion agrees that it is a rotatory movement about an oblique axis.

von Meyer (1853) appears to have been the first investigator to state clearly that the talus rotates on the calcaneus about an oblique axis. This was confirmed by Henke (1855, 1863) and by Meyer (1883) in his book entitled *Studien über den Mechanismus des Fusses*, with the statement, "*dass die Bewegung des Astragalus gegenüber der übrigen Fusswurzel um eine schief liegende Axe zu Stande kommt, welche von der inneren Seite der oberen Fläche des Astragalus-Halses in die Mitte des unteren Randes der hinteren Fläche des Kalkaneus geht.*" Two line drawings accompany this statement and clearly depict the position of the axis as projected upon the transverse and sagittal planes. However, there appeared even at this early date a disagreement as to whether the rotation of the talus upon the calcaneus was merely rotation over conical surfaces (Meyer) or was accompanied by a forward and backward displacement of the talus along the axis (a screwlike movement). Henke (1863) maintained that the rotation of the calcaneus about the oblique axis of the talus is definitely screwlike: "*eine am linken Fusse linksgewundene Schraubenbewegung.*" Dönitz (1903) exhaustively studied the motion between the talus and the calcaneus, employing six different techniques to gather his data, and arrived at the conclusion that the motion is a rotatory one about a single axis; however, he leaves unanswered the specific question of whether the rotation is screwlike, with a spatial displacement of the bones forward and backward along the axis. Fick (1904) agreed with Henke that the motion was essentially screwlike. Elftman and Manter (1935) reviewed the literature and accepted the findings of the previous investigators that movement between the two bones was about an oblique axis but did not attempt to answer the question of whether or not this rotation was accompanied by a longitudinal displacement of the talus upon the calcaneus (screwlike motion). Manter (1941) carefully studied the motion in the subtalar joint in 16 cadaver specimens. He reported the average inclination of the axis of the subtalar joint to be 42° projected onto the sagittal plane and deviating anteriorly and medially by 16° in the horizontal plane from a line connecting the midpoint of the heel to the interval between the first and second toes.

Isman and Inman (1968), using a modification of Manter's optical method of locating the axis, reported measurements on 46 cadaver feet. Their average angles, as projected onto the horizontal and vertical planes, agreed precisely with those of Manter, but there was a greater range of individual variation. While Manter employed the interval between the first and second matatarsals as his base line for measuring the angulation of the axis in the horizontal plane, Isman and Inman employed the midline of the foot, which resulted in a slightly larger angle by approximately 6 to 8°. The study by Isman and Inman was extended to include angular measurements on 56 additional specimens without any significant differences in the mean values or the standard deviations (Appendix F). The inclination of the axis as projected onto a vertical (sagittal) plane was 42° ± 9° (Fig. 9.1) and its deviation from the midline of the foot in a horizontal plane was 23° ± 11° (Fig. 9.2). However, it should be noted that while the average values for the inclination and medial deviation of the axis of the subtalar joint are remarkably close, there exists a wide difference among individuals. Manter in his series stated that the "amount of vertical tilt varied between 29 and 47 degrees," and the "medial slant" varied between 8 and 24°. In Isman and Inman's and

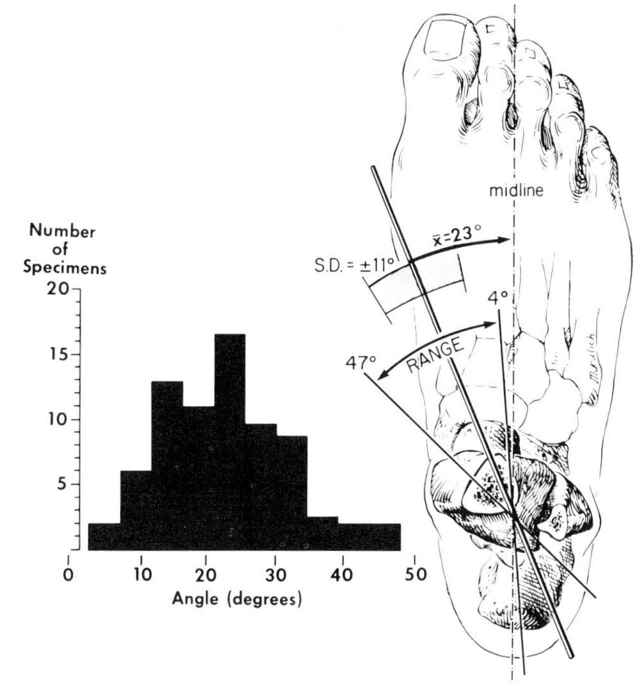

FIG. 9.2. Variations in position of subtalar axis as projected onto transverse plane. The angle was measured between the axis and the midline of the foot. The extent of individual variation is shown on the *sketch* and revealed in the *histogram*.

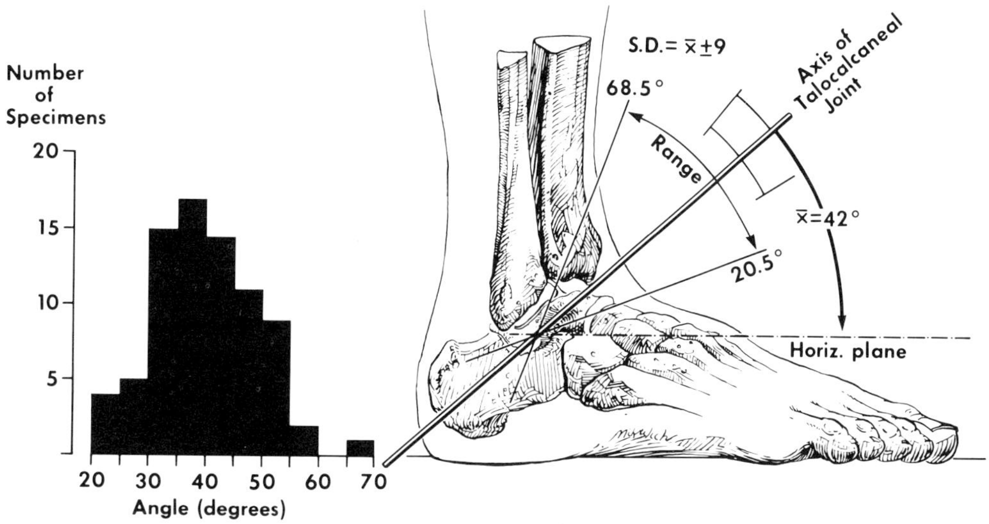

FIG. 9.1. Variations in inclination of axis of subtalar joint as projected upon sagittal plane. The distribution of the measurements on the individual specimens is shown in the *histogram*. The single observation of an angle of almost 70° was present in a markedly cavus foot.

in our series the variation was found to be between 20 and 68° for the inclination of the axis in the sagittal plane and between 4 and 47° in the amount of medial deviation.

In summary, it now appears well established that motion between the talus and the calcaneus is a rotatory one about a single oblique axis. The action of the talocalcaneal joint may therefore be likened to that of a "mitered hinge" (see Fig. 9.3) connecting the leg to the foot. Within a limited range, longitudinal rotation of the leg imposes a longitudinal rotation of the foot (supination and pronation). For more details, see Chapter 11, "Biomechanics of the Subtalar Joint."

While the analogy between the subtalar joint and a mitered hinge depicts accurately the basic type of linkage that is present between the talus and the calcaneus, it fails to include certain additional anatomic and functional factors that have been postulated in the literature. For the sake of completeness and possible clinical importance these factors must be discussed in some detail.

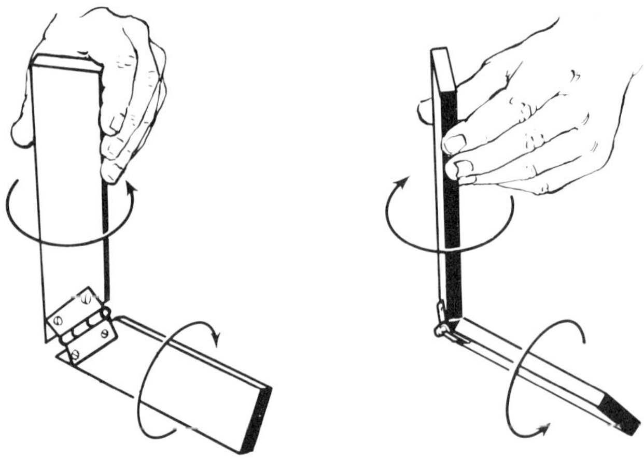

FIG. 9.3. Representation of subtalar joint as mitered hinge connecting leg (vertical member) to foot (horizontal member). Rotation of one member results in rotation of the other member. In the living, internal and external rotation of the leg causes pronation and supination of the foot.(from Inman, Verne T., and Mann, Roger A. Biomechanics of the foot and ankle. In Inman, V. T. (ed.) *DuVries' Surgery of the Foot*. Ed. 3, The C. V. Mosby Co., St. Louis, 1973).

QUESTION OF THE SCREWLIKE MOTION OF THE SUBTALAR JOINT

As noted in the literature review, several investigators have maintained that the rotation of the talus upon the calcaneus is accompanied by a longitudinal displacement of the bones along the axis of rotation. The motion would therefore resemble that of a screw. Manter (1941) was the most specific. He calculated an average helix angle of 12° and stated that the head of the talus moves forward in pronation and that "its forward displacement would be approximately 1.5 mm. for each 10 degrees of rotation in the subtalar joint." If this is true, the forward displacement of the talus might carry the malleoli with it, assuming there is no other compensating mechanism such as a more distal attachment of the ligament. While the effect upon the medial collateral ligament and upon the posterior and anterior talofibular ligaments would be negligible, the calcaneofibular ligament, which extends across the subtalar joint, might be subjected to increasing or decreasing tension with movement of the subtalar joint. Since Manter reported only an average value obtained from 16 specimens, the screwlike motion between the talus and the calcaneus seemed to require a more detailed investigation.

Two studies on 42 and 102 cadaver specimens (Appendix F) and an additional roentgenographic investigation of 50 dry bones (Appendix I) were carried out with the hope of shedding more light upon the subject of the screwlike motion between the talus and the calcaneus.

Contouring the Posterior Calcaneal Facet

Since the posterior facet appears to be the sole factor that dictates whether or not the talus migrates on the calcaneus forward or backward along the empirical axis with movement of the subtalar joint, the posterior facet of the calcaneus was contoured with a dial indicator (Appendix F). If the posterior facet exhibited the properties of a screw, then with rotation of the calcaneus the dial indicator should reveal progressively changing values. A true screw would show constant increments of longitudinal displacement with each degree of rotation and would require continuing congruence between the articulating surfaces throughout the motion. In this study the statement of Huson (1961) was verified, that true congruence occurred only in the midposition of the joint; some degree of incongruence was apparent at the extremes of motion. It is apparent that the posterior articulation of the talocalcaneal joint is not a precisely lapped machine-like joint, but it was felt that the incongruence was not sufficiently great to affect the validity of the studies.

The entire surface of the posterior facet was contoured. This was possible because of the small size of the contact point on the arm of the dial indicator, and it resulted in an extent of rotation in excess of that permitted normally between the talus and the calcaneus. The articular surfaces were contoured at 5-

and 10-mm distances from the axial rod. Specimens from right and left feet were rotated in opposite directions so that the deflections on the dial indicator would be comparable. The contours extended from the medial to the lateral edge of the articular surface. While the contour lines made at the 5-mm distance tended generally to follow the 10-mm lines, they were shorter and more irregular. Therefore they were not used for quantitation. Typical curves of individual specimens are reproduced in Appendix F. The marked variation from specimen to specimen should be noted. Obviously, the accuracy of location of the axis would influence these measurements.

If the posterior facet exhibits the characteristics of a screw, the curves relating rotation of the calcaneus in degrees to the linear displacement as recorded by the dial indicator should be a straight line. The slope of the line indicates the pitch of the screw. It was found that approximately one-half of the specimens could be considered screwlike, as depicted by the reasonably straight curves, which, however, had varying pitches. The remainder were very unscrewlike in their behavior. Some initially moved in one direction, only to reverse themselves later. Others started in the opposite direction but as the rotation progressed, they also reversed their direction. A few showed pure rotation with no linear displacement. The data on the 42 specimens are summarized in Figure 9.4.

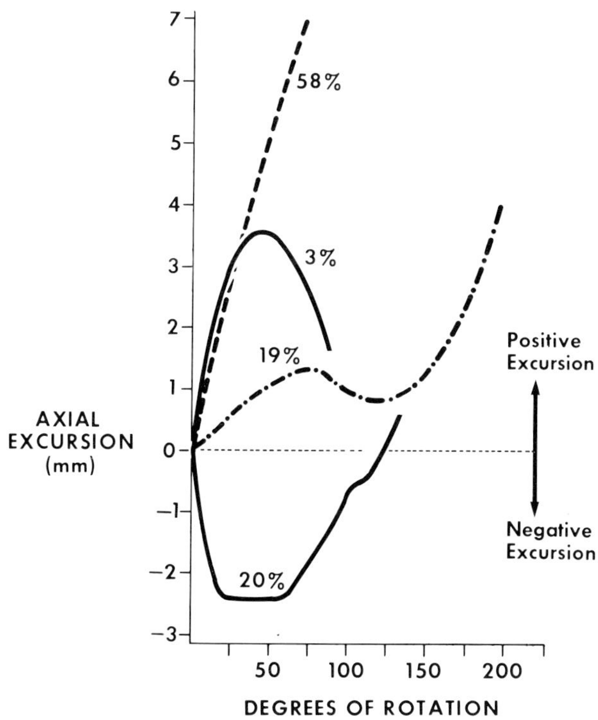

FIG. 9.4. Graphical summary of data from contouring of posterior facet of calcaneus. Precise values should not be taken from these curves since they are only summary curves of grouped measurements. Examples of individual measurements are shown in Appendix F. Note that a little more than half of the specimens (58%) show constant increments of axial excursion indicating a screwlike motion. The remainder of the specimens behaved in a variety of unscrewlike ways.

Since the slopes of the curves of those specimens which demonstrated a screwlike motion varied and since nearly half of the specimens were very unscrewlike, the calculation of an average helix angle or pitch would appear to be more misleading than illuminating. Such an average value might be assumed to represent a so-called normal situation which exists in all feet. This is not true. The remarkable variation is the important factor, and a realization of the existence of these variations is important in any functional evaluation of the foot.

Linear Displacement of the Talus on the Calcaneus

Since the talar facet, which constitutes the other half of the articulation, was ignored in the previous study, it was realized that contouring the posterior facet of the calcaneus may not have completely answered the question of longitudinal displacement of the talus along the empirical axis with movement of the subtalar joint. Therefore the displacement was measured directly with the talus and the calcaneus articulated (Appendix F). With the dial indicator mounted in line with the axis and the calcaneus firmly fixed, the talus was rotated. Any forward or backward movement could be recorded directly from the readings on the dial indicator. The study, which included the 42 specimens of the preceding investigation, was expanded to 102 specimens. A summary of the results of this study indicates that only slightly over one-half (58 of 102) of the specimens demonstrated an absolute linear displacement of the talus forward on the axis of the subtalar joint as this joint was rotated from a position of full supination to full pronation. It is interesting to note that this occurred more frequently on the right side (34 of 48) than on the left side (24 of 54). At the present time no comment can be made on this finding. The remaining specimens demonstrated (1) no excursion, (2) negative excursions, or (3) complex movements similar to the contour curves shown in Figure 9.4.

Of those specimens which showed progressive linear displacements, only 20 of the 102 specimens showed relatively constant increments and therefore could be considered essentially screwlike. For these, the average pitch was calculated out of pure curiosity. This was found to be 1.12 cm, or two-thirds as great as reported by Manter (1.7 cm) and approximately one-half of the value of the pitch (2.08 cm) calculated from the curvature of the posterior articular facet of the calcaneus on the same 20 specimens. This indicated that the actual linear displacement when measured directly was somewhat less than that revealed by the contouring of the posterior facet of the calcaneus alone. Therefore the talar half of the subtalar articulation in these specimens had a diminishing effect upon the actual linear displacement of the talus on the calcaneus with movement of the subtalar joint.

X-ray Studies on Dry Bones

Fifty matched pairs of tali and calcanei in which the axis of the subtalar joint had been determined in another investigation were available for study (Appendix I). X-rays of each articulated talus and calcaneus were taken with the beam perpendicular to the plane of the axis. In the films the projection of the posterior articulation of the talus and the calcaneus was plainly visible as a discrete and almost straight crevice (Fig. 9.5). Therefore it appeared reasonable to assume that the angle between a perpendicular dropped from the axis line and the line representing the plane of the joint could be considered to approximate the helix angle (Fig. 9.6). This angle was measured in 50 specimens. The average was 25° ± 6°, with a range of 0 to 40°.

The average helix angle measured in the x-ray studies of 50 dried bony specimens was twice that reported by Manter on 16 cadaver specimens. Taken alone these findings would certainly support the contention that the motion of the talus upon the calcaneus must be screwlike. However, attention should be called to the marked individual differences, which varied from a zero helix angle to one of 40°. Furthermore, the conclusion that movement is screwlike—based solely upon the data obtained from measuring the inclination of the posterior facet of the calcaneus—appears unjustified, since the measurements from contouring the articular surface of the posterior facet and the direct measurement of the linear displacement of the talus along the axis of the subtalar joint (see above) do not support such an unqualified deduction.

While the investigators were puzzling over a possible explanation for the wide variability in the angle of the posterior facet of the subtalar joint and the empirical axis as measured on the x-rays of the dried bony specimens, an interesting observation was made. The crevice denoting the posterior articulation appeared always to lie at a right angle to the trabeculae

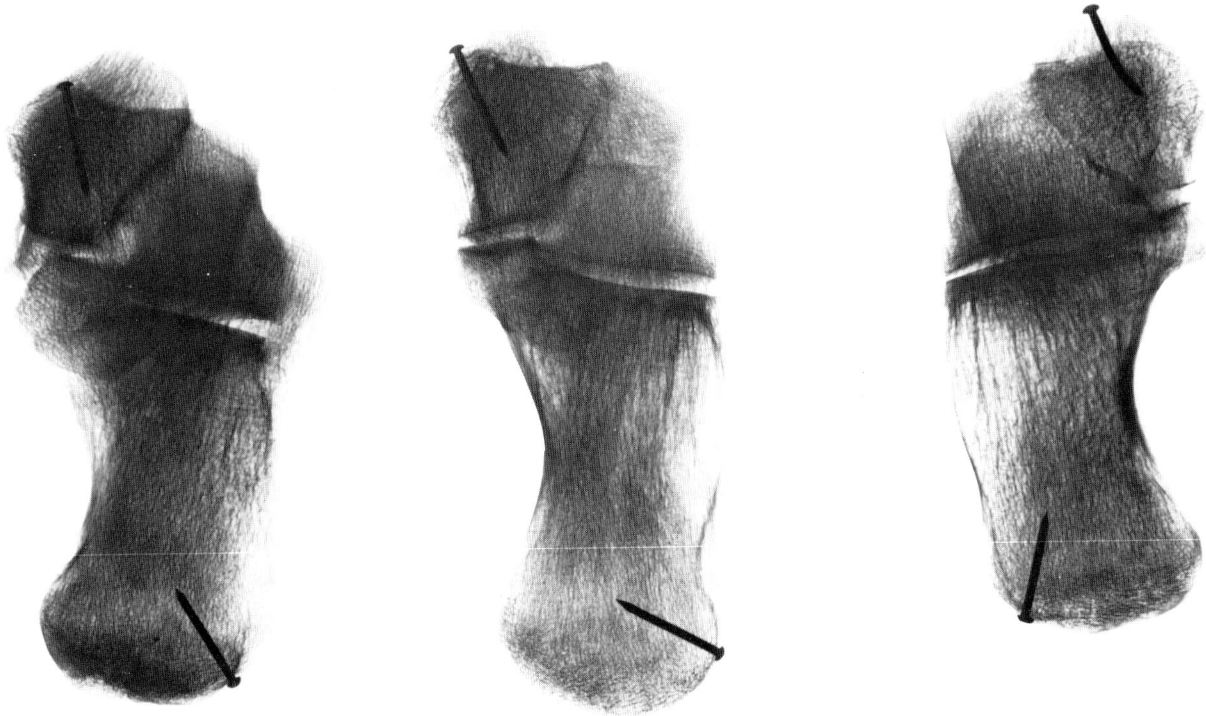

FIG. 9.5. Dorsiplantar x-rays of three randomly selected specimens of dried tali and calcanei. The straight crevice of the joint is clearly visible. Note that the trabeculae of the calcanei tend to become parallel as they approach the posterior facet and that the joint surface is oriented to lie perpendicular to these trabeculae.

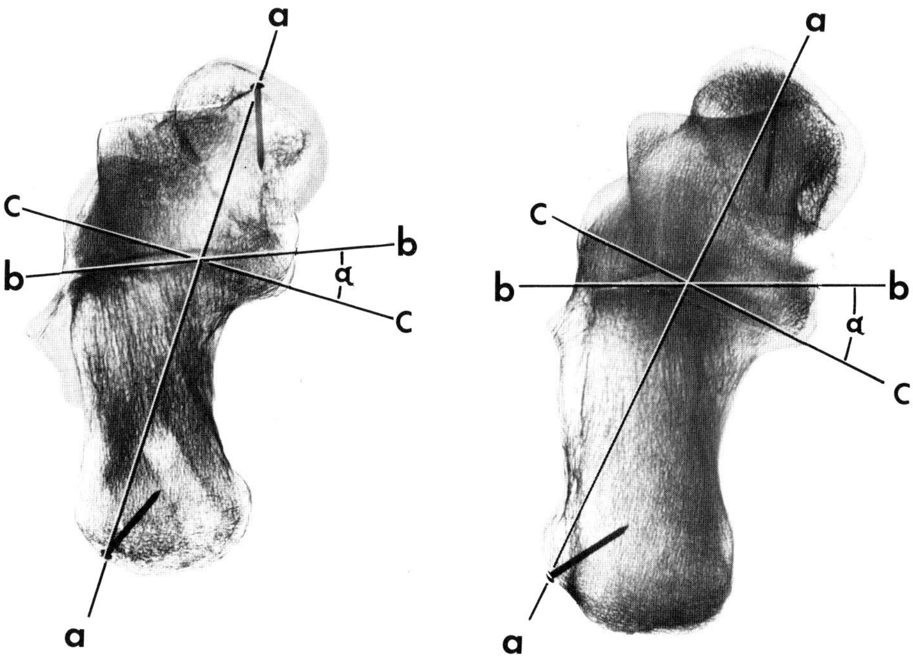

FIG. 9.6. Measurement of presumed helix angle. *Line a*——a, connecting the escutcheon pins, locates the axis of the subtalar joint. *Line b*——b is drawn to overlie and parallel the posterior articulation of the subtalar joint. *Line c*——c is drawn at a right angle to line a——a. The angle α is the presumed helix angle.

of the calcaneus, which tended to become parallel as they approached the joint surface. This is clearly shown in Figure 9.5. To verify this casual observation the angle between the posterior facet and a line drawn parallel to the trabeculae was measured in the 50 specimens. The average angle was 92° ± 5°, with a maximal range of 80 to 100°. The coefficient of variation was small (5.79%) (Fig. 9.7)

Unfortunately, when this study was carried out lateral x-rays of only six of the 50 bony specimens were secured. However, in these few specimens the superior group of trabeculae were seen to lie almost perpendicular to the joint surface (see Fig. 9.8). The following conclusions seem warranted from these observations. In the transverse plane the orientation of the posterior facet of the subtalar joint is nearly always perpendicular to the bony trabeculae. In the sagittal plane this also appears to be true but this is only an impression and is unsupported by adequate data.

If the trabeculae are assumed to depict the lines of compressive forces in the bone, then a reasonable explanation for the orientation of the joint surfaces is suggested. The posterior facet of the subtalar joint is so located that the major forces are compressive forces acting perpendicularly to the joint surfaces. In such a situation the joint would always be free to move under load since tangential forces must be small. Therefore,

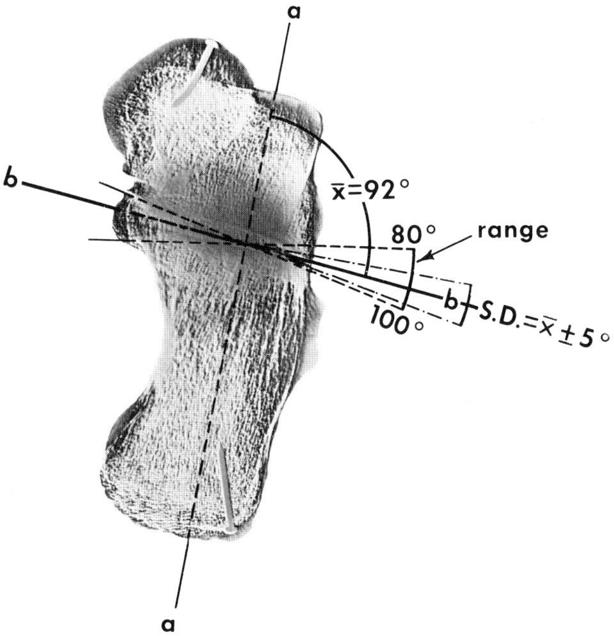

FIG. 9.7. Results of angular measurements between trabeculae of calcaneus and articular surface of posterior facet of subtalar joint in 50 dried bony specimens. *Line a*——a was drawn by eye to parallel the trabeculae. *Line b*——b parallels the joint.

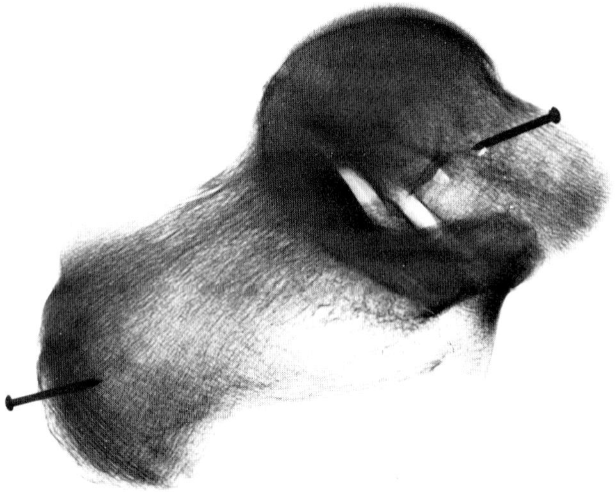

FIG. 9.8. Lateral x-ray of articulated talus and calcaneus. Note that the trabeculae approach the posterior articular facet of the calcaneus at a right angle to the articular surface.

it appears that the precise orientation of a joint is more dependent upon the intrinsic forces transmitted to the joint surfaces than upon the axis of motion. Variations in the individual shapes of the calcanei and tali are obvious and must reflect genetic and developmental factors. These must affect the trabecular pattern and in turn the orientation of the joint. Support for such a conclusion is based upon the constancy of the relationship that obtains between the trabecular pattern in the calcaneus and the joint surface.

These observations suggest that the final positioning of the posterior articulation of the subtalar joint is influenced more by the intrinsic forces acting through the joint than by its axis of motion. Such a conclusion might explain the marked variability found in the actual behavior of the joint.

RANGES OF MOTION AT THE SUBTALAR JOINT

As previously suggested in the text, the talocrural and talocalcaneal joints should be considered together as a functional unit. There is evidence that the two articulations may act in a complementary manner during locomotion. Since there is little specific information in the literature on the ranges of motion permitted in the subtalar joint, it was felt necessary to undertake an investigation both on cadaver material and on living subjects. Two studies on cadaver specimens and one on living subjects were completed (Appendix J). As was to be expected, wide variations in the amount of motion were found. In the cadaver material the ranges of motion varied from 10 to 59°. The averages differed in the various series depending on the technique employed. In one series of 47 specimens, with ligaments intact, the average was 18° ± 6°, and in the same series with all ligaments removed, the range of motion was doubled, with an average of 36° ± 10°. The values obtained from the 102 specimens employed in the study of the screwlike motion of the subtalar joint gave an average of 24° ± 11°. In 50 living subjects (100 ankles) the average motion was 40° ± 7°, with a range of 20 to 65°, as measured with the spherical goniometer (see Appendix J).

The differences in the average values of the range of motion of the subtalar joint obtained from the various studies may at first glance be somewhat disconcerting. However, these differences merely emphasize the irrationality of thinking solely in terms of averages. The important fact is the wide variability; motion in the subtalar joint may vary from 10 to 65°. This fact should be kept clearly in mind when the foot of any single individual is examined.

SUMMARY

Movement between the talus and the calcaneus consists of rotation about a single oblique axis. In general, the axis extends from the neck of the talus downward and laterally through the sinus tarsi and emerges on the lateral side of the calcaneus. While the average inclination as projected onto the sagittal plane approximates 42° to the plantar surface of the foot, there are wide individual variations. The axis may be more horizontal—in extreme cases forming an angle of only 22°—or more vertical, with an angle of as much as 68° (see Fig. 9.1). Furthermore, the position of the axis as projected onto a transverse plane also varies considerably from its average value of 23° (see Fig. 9.2). The effects of these variations will be discussed in the section on biomechanics.

The answer to the question of whether or not rotation between the talus and the calcaneus is accompanied by a linear displacement along the axis of movement (screwlike motion) requires a certain delimitation. It appears reasonable to assume that in approximately one-half of the population there is some linear displacement of the talus along the axis with movement in the subtalar joint. In this context, the motion may be considered screwlike; however, the pitch of the screw varies widely from individual to individual. In the other half of the population the motion is very unscrewlike and the talus may or may not be displaced forward or backward with movement between the talus and the calcaneus. While great variability is found in the orientation of the posterior facet to the axis of movement and in the behavior of the joint on motion, there appears to be a definite and precise relationship between the articular surfaces and the trabecular pattern in the calcaneus.

The range of motion of the subtalar joint has been shown to vary markedly within the population. In cadaver material and in the living, a range of motion of 10 to 60° was found.

Introduction to Chapters 10 and 11

The ankle joint and the subtalar joint, taken together, have been likened to a universal coupling connecting the leg and the calcaneus (Wright *et al.*, 1964). This analogy is only accurate when specific relationships exist. A true universal coupling (or cardan joint) requires two swivel pins to be set at 90° to one another. This never occurs between the axes of the ankle and the subtalar joints. The transmission of the rotatory motions between leg and calcaneus, therefore, is variable and complex. The final effect depends upon the specific orientation of the two axes in each individual. Before attempting to develop a quantitative relationship, which involves several variables, it seems appropriate to discuss qualitatively the effects of the variations in orientation of these axes. For the sake of clarity of presentation, the results of variations in orientation of the axes of the ankle and subtalar joints will be considered separately. In each situation the joint under discussion will be assumed to be the sole connection between the leg and the foot, and the entire foot will be depicted as a single rigid structure.

The biomechanics of the ankle joint will be discussed first. This will be followed by a discussion of the biomechanics of the subtalar joint. Finally, the interaction between the two articulations will be discussed in a qualitative manner.

10

Biomechanics of the Ankle Joint

Since detailed written descriptions can become so involved and mathematical presentations so abstruse as to be ineffectual in transmitting to the reader a clear understanding of the consequences of the variability in the position of the axis of the ankle, it has been decided to utilize a simple model in an attempt to depict these effects. It is realized that the employment of such a simplistic presentation of the ankle will not accurately reproduce the true anatomic conditions that exist in any single individual. However, certain basic relationships are clearly made more understandable.

In the model, the ankle will be considered a single-axis joint and will be represented by a hinge. The leg consists of a vertical wooden member. The foot is considered to be a rigid structure and is shown as a wooden piece, roughly shaped to resemble the outline of the foot. The midline of the foot is indicated by a black line on its dorsal and plantar surfaces. The hinge is the only connecting element between the leg and the foot. Fastened to the foot is a plastic disk, which is calibrated in 10° increments. The basic model to be employed represents a right leg and foot and is shown in Figure 10.1. Subsequent models will reveal the effects of varying the position of the hinge in the coronal and in the transverse planes. To emphasize these effects, the selected positions of the hinge in the models are those that represent extreme values as determined from the anthropometric studies. It should be obvious to the reader that the employment of average values will produce similar results, but the effects will be less apparent. The assumption has been made that exaggeration, used in moderation, contributes to good pedagogy.

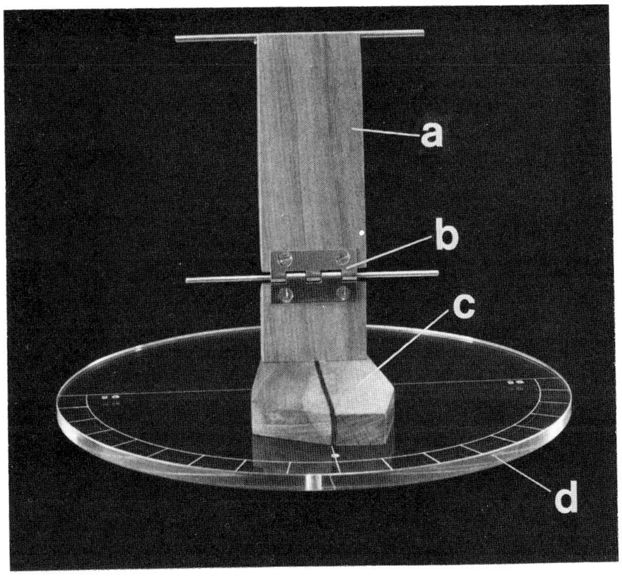

FIG. 10.1. Photograph of basic model to be used in demonstrating effects of variations in position of ankle axis. The vertical wooden member (*a*) represents the leg. It carries on its upper end a short metal rod that represents the axis of the knee joint. The hinge (*b*) represents the ankle joint. The pin of the hinge has been extended for easier reference. The foot (*c*) is represented by a horizontal wooden member roughly shaped to resemble a right foot and is attached to the ankle hinge by a short vertical piece. The midline of the foot is shown as a black line. Fixed to the foot is a plastic disk (*d*) calibrated in 10° increments from the zero position, which is the sagittal plane of the foot and leg. The inscribed diameter of the disk that connects the two 90° calibrations will always be kept in the same vertical plane as the knee axis. The amount of toeing in or toeing out can be determined by noting the position of the black line on the foot in relation to the calibrations on the disk.

For simplicity of presentation, the photographs of the models will be grouped into two series. The first series assumes that the leg is fixed in space while the foot is free to move in directions dictated by the orientation of the hinge. In the second series the foot is assumed to be fixed on the ground and immobile; the effects of the different orientations of the ankle axis in the latter series will therefore be upon the leg and not upon the foot.

FOOT FREE, LEG FIXED

Variable Position of the Ankle Axis in Relation to the Knee Axis in the Transverse Plane

As pointed out in the section on tibial or malleolar torsion in Chapter 3, "The Axis of the Ankle Joint," p.8, the presumed axis of the knee joint has been utilized as the reference plane to measure the variations in the position of the ankle axis as projected onto a transverse plane. The averages reported by most investigators are comparable and approximate 23° of "external tibial torsion" in adults; that is, the axis of the ankle is inclined laterally and posteriorly in relation to the knee axis by that amount. However, the individual angular differences between the two axes have been demonstrated to be exceedingly great. The reported extremes on either side of the mean may exceed 30°. The basic model is modified by the insertion of a pivot just above the ankle hinge to permit the hinged ankle joint with its attached foot to be rotated laterally and medially from a midposition. The hinge retains a constant position of 90° to the midline of the foot. The leg, represented by the vertical wooden structure, remains in a fixed position in space, while the ankle hinge with its foot is varied to positions of 25° of "internal" and "external" torsion. The plane of plantar flexion and dorsiflexion of the ankle is clearly revealed when the circular transparent plastic disk is observed. A "Devil Level,"* fixed to the foot and aligned at a right angle to the midline of the foot, is utilized to demonstrate any rotatory displacements of the foot that may occur about its long axis with plantar flexion and dorsiflexion of the ankle. Three views have been employed, one in the midposition, one in 20° of dorsiflexion, and one in 30° of plantar flexion. Rather than having the reader attempt to follow an extensive verbal description in the text, it is suggested that each set of photographs will call the reader's attention to the pertinent effects (Figs. 10.2 and 10.3).

In summary, the models demonstrate that if the axis of the hinge remains horizontal and in a fixed position of 90° to the midline of the foot, dorsiflexion and plantar flexion of the ankle produce no rotation of

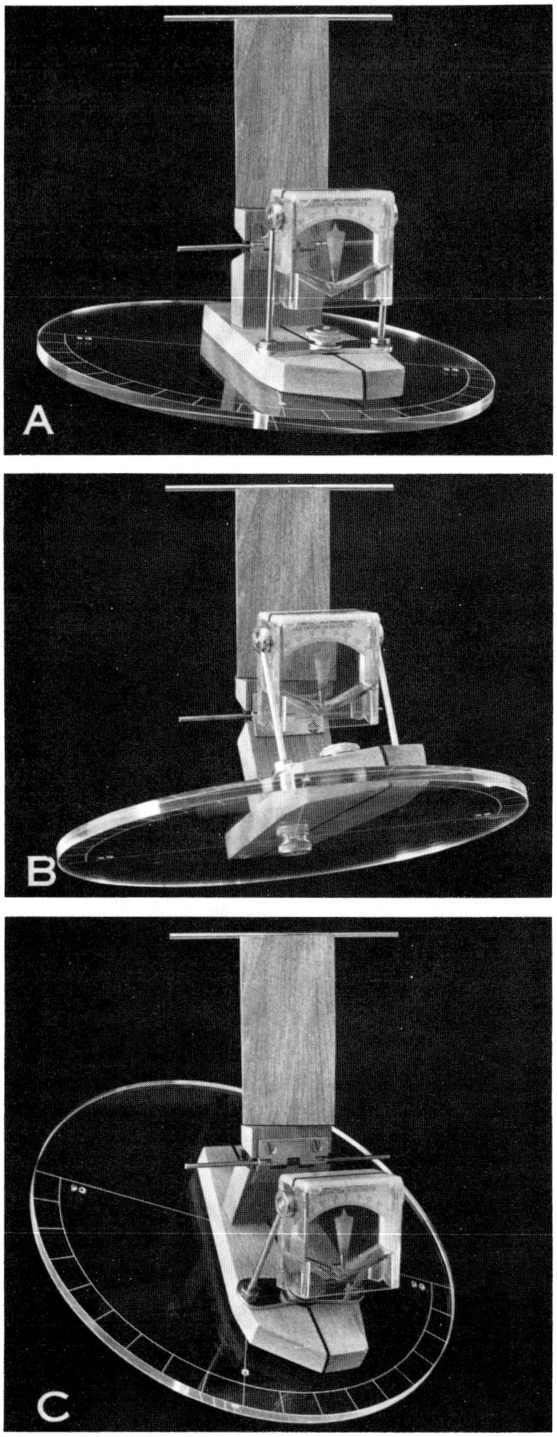

FIGURE 10.2

* A commercially available instrument that measures, directly in degrees, the changes in inclination from the horizontal plane (Pickett Industries, Inc., Santa Barbara, California).

the foot about its long axis (midline). Dorsiflexion and plantar flexion occur in a vertical plane, but this plane deviates from the sagittal plane by the amount of horizontal displacement of the ankle axis in relation to the knee axis. The foot is simply toed in or toed out during its entire motion of dorsiflexion and plantar flexion.

Variable Position of the Ankle Axis in Relation to the Midline of the Foot in the Transverse Plane

The majority of textbooks of anatomy in which the position of the ankle axis is discussed, state that the ankle axis is directed laterally and posteriorly in relation to the midline of the foot when referred onto a horizontal plane. Anthropometric studies (Isman and Inman, 1968) on cadaver specimens confirmed this finding. The average deviation of the ankle axis from the midline of the foot was found to be in the vicinity of 6°. However, individual variations occur. Instances of anterolateral deviations were found that were in excess of 20°, while in a few specimens the angle between the midline of the foot and the axis of the ankle joint was reversed and was found to be directed laterally and anteriorly by a few degrees.

The effect of changing the angular relationships between the axis of the ankle joint and the midline of the foot is revealed in photographs of the model. For simplicity of presentation the axis, the knee joint, and the ankle hinge in this series of photographs remain in a fixed parallel position. Only the foot will be rotated medially or laterally in relationship to the ankle hinge (Figs. 10.4 and 10.5).

It will be noted from a study of the photographs that deviations from the one position where the long axis—midline—of the foot is at a right angle to the ankle cause a rotation of the foot about its long axis

FIG. 10.2. Series of photographs of model in Figure 10.1, showing ankle hinge with its attached foot rotated medially 25° in relation to knee axis. The diameter inscribed on the plastic disk, connecting the 90° marks, remains in the plane of the knee axis. The medial rotation of the foot of 25° is readily seen by relating the position of the black line on the foot to the inscribed 10° increments on the plastic disk. The ankle hinge is at a right angle to the midline of the foot and the Devil Level remains parallel to the ankle hinge. The vertical plane of motion dictated by the ankle hinge is now no longer in the sagittal plane of the leg but in a new vertical plane rotated medially by 25° from the knee axis. From the neutral position (*A*), the model is dorsiflexed 20° (*B*), and plantar flexed 30° (*C*). The following particulars should be noted. The plane of movement is now oblique to the coronal plane as determined by the knee axis. The plane of movement as depicted by the plastic disk and projected onto the coronal plane appears to tilt on dorsiflexion and plantar flexion of the foot. However, the Devil Level, which remains parallel to the ankle axis, reveals that no rotation of the foot about its long axis occurs.

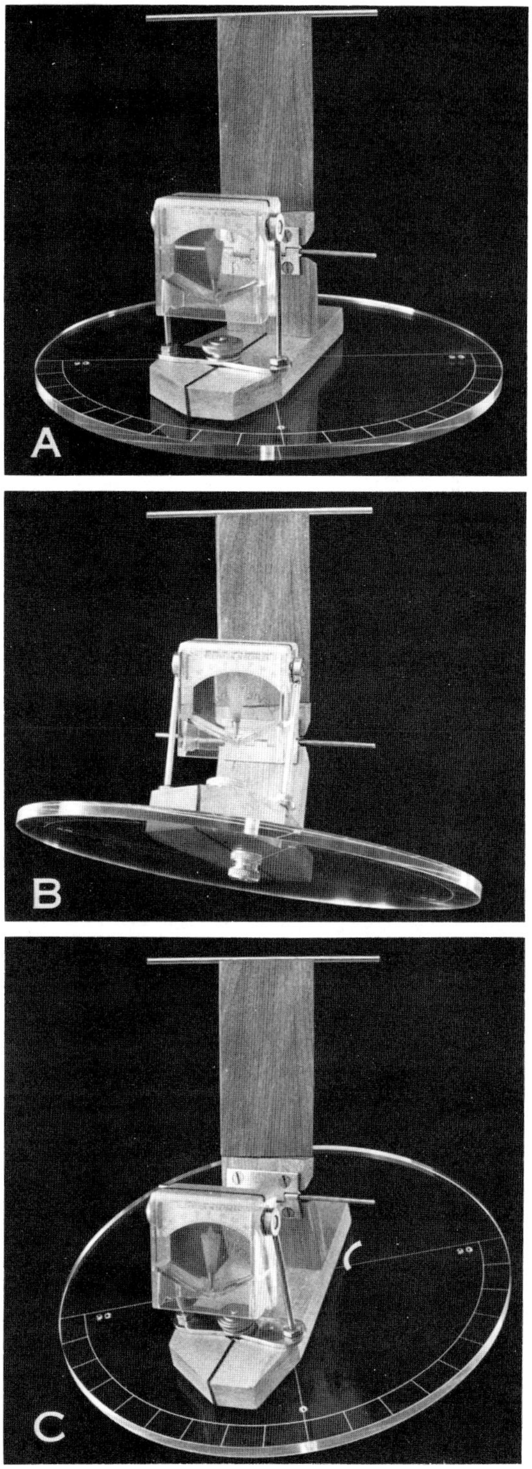

FIG. 10.3. Effect of rotating foot of model laterally 25° in relation to knee axis. Again note that dorsiflexion (*B*) and plantar flexion (*C*) of the foot occur in a vertical plane that is oblique to the sagittal plane of the leg. The inclinations of the plastic disk are reversed from those in Figure 10.2, but there is still no rotation of the foot about its long axis as revealed by the Devil Level. The foot is simply dorsiflexing and plantar flexing in a plane that is oblique to the sagittal plane of the leg.

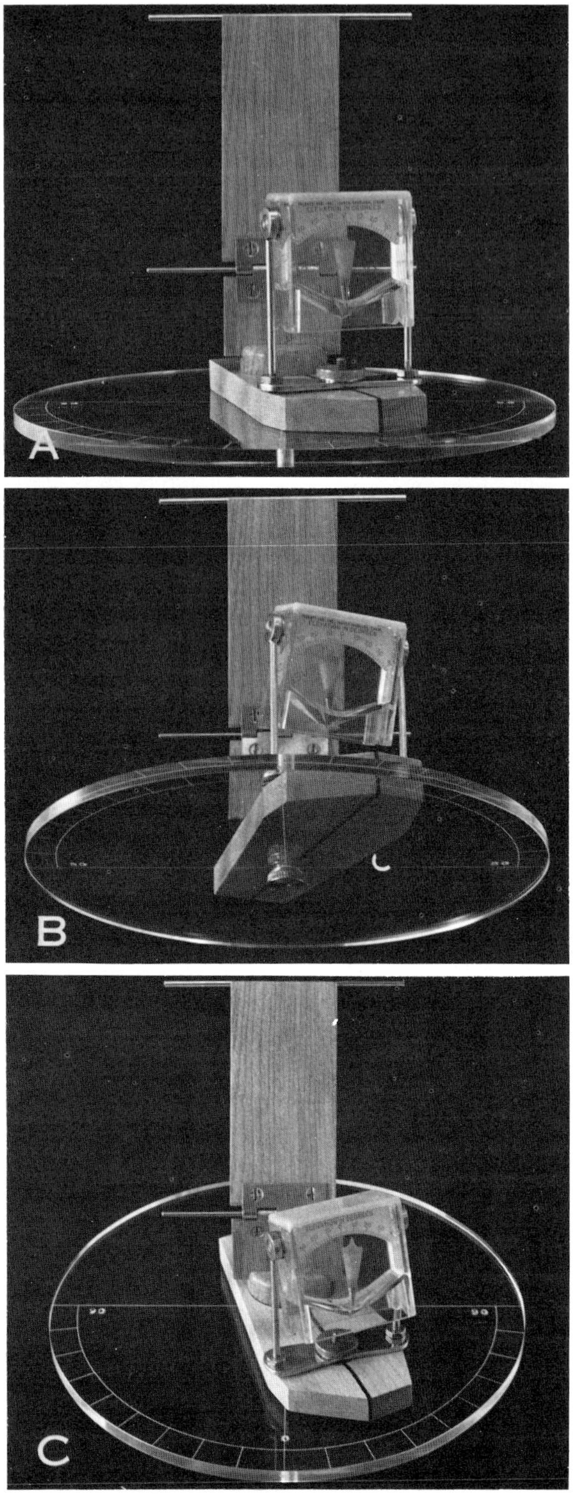

FIG. 10.4. Ankle (hinge) and knee axes parallel and in same vertical (coronal) plane. The foot has been rotated medially 25° to the coronal plane of the ankle hinge. Attention is directed to the Devil Level, which shows that in dorsiflexion (*B*) and plantar flexion (*C*) there is rotation of the foot about its long axis. The direction of this rotation on dorsiflexion is a pronatory one. The longitudinal rotation in plantar flexion is in a reverse direction (supinatory).

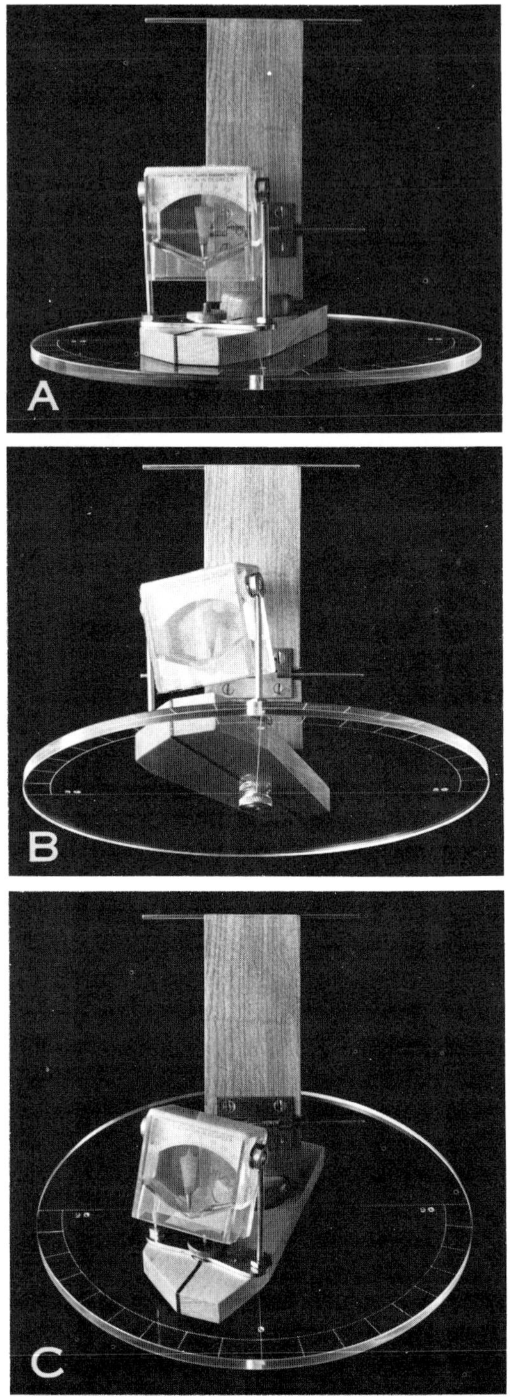

FIG. 10.5. Same projections of model as in Figure 10.4. The foot, however, has been rotated laterally in relation to the ankle axis by 25°. Reference to the Devil Level demonstrates that again there is a rotation of the foot about its long axis on dorsiflexion and plantar flexion. The direction of this rotation is opposite to that shown in Figure 10.4.

with dorsiflexion and plantar flexion of the ankle. The amount of this rotation of the foot will vary as the sine of the angle of deviation of the foot from the sagittal plane of the leg.

Variable Position of the Ankle Axis in the Coronal Plane

As previously discussed, the axis of the ankle joint is rarely if ever horizontal when projected onto the coronal plane. It is inclined downward from the medial to the lateral side. The degree of obliquity varies; the average inclination is 12°, with a maximal inclination of 23°. The effect of an oblique inclination of the ankle axis is shown in the next series of photographs of the wooden model. The ankle hinge is oriented downward and laterally at an angle of 23° with the leg. In Figure 10.6 the ankle hinge, while inclined 23° in a vertical plane, remains parallel to the knee axis and at a right angle to the midline of the foot. Dorsiflexion and plantar flexion about this obliquely placed hinge produce no longitudinal rotation but do cause the foot to toe out on dorsiflexion and toe in on plantar flexion. This is not so apparent in the photographs of the model since the amounts of dorsiflexion (20°) and plantar flexion (30°) are small. In Figure 10.7 the plastic disk and the Devil Level have been removed from the model and the extent of flexion and extension has been increased to 40° of both dorsiflexion and plantar flexion. The amounts of toeing out on dorsiflexion and toeing in on plantar flexion are now obvious.

Effect of Combining the Axial Positions in the Transverse and Coronal Planes

In the living person, the ankle axis is obliquely oriented in both the transverse and coronal planes when related to the foot. From the medial to the lateral side, the axis is inclined backward and downward. This situation is depicted in the next series of photographs of the model (Figs. 10.8 and 10.9), which combine the separate axial positions presented in the previous photographs.

It was hoped that some correlation existed between the orientation of the axis of the ankle in the two planes of space, but scatter diagrams of the individual angular values obtained from 46 cadaver feet revealed no evidence of correlation. At present it appears that the degree of obliquity of the ankle in the coronal plane and the amount that it deviates from the midline of the foot in the transverse plane are independent variables. The effects of the two inclinations can be separated. A review of the models indicates that angular deviations in the transverse

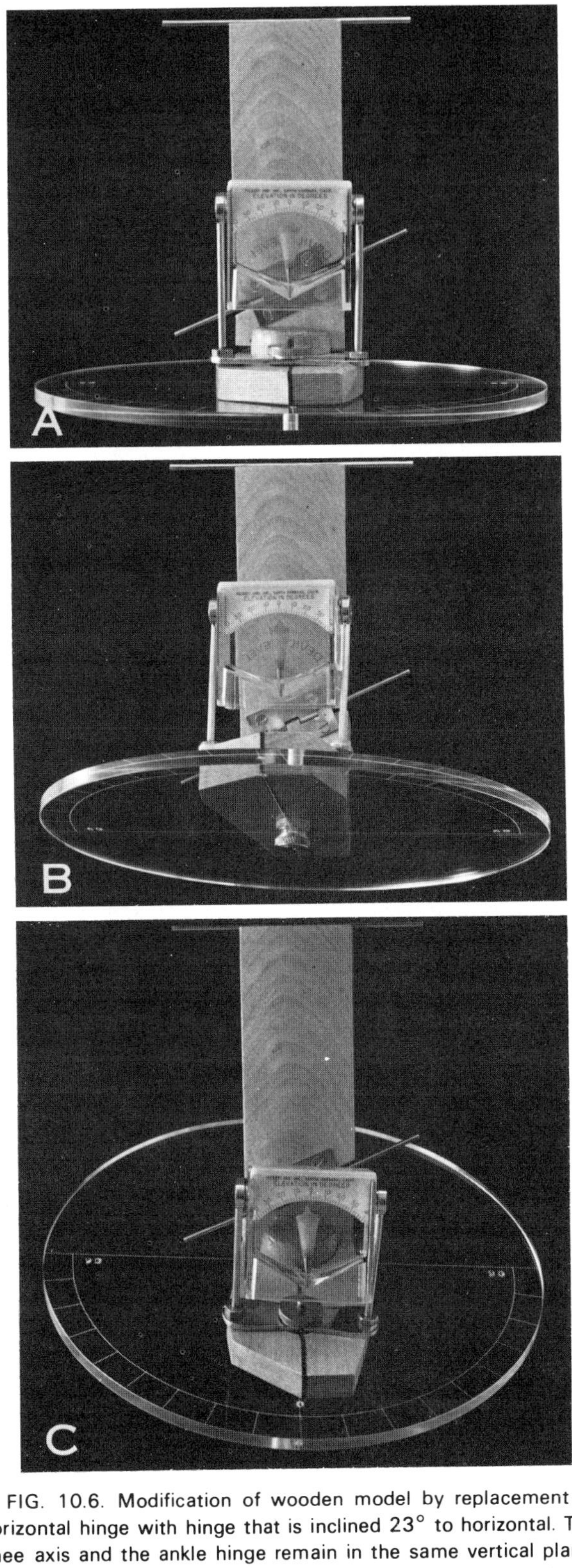

FIG. 10.6. Modification of wooden model by replacement of horizontal hinge with hinge that is inclined 23° to horizontal. The knee axis and the ankle hinge remain in the same vertical plane. The midline of the foot is at a right angle to this plane. Attention is directed to the Devil Level. Note that on dorsiflexion and on plantar flexion there is little longitudinal rotation of the foot about its long axis. The foot toes slightly outward on dorsiflexion (*B*) and slightly inward on plantar flexion (*C*).

plane, from the single position in which the midline of the foot and the ankle axis are at a right angle, cause longitudinal rotations of the foot with flexion and extension (pronatory and supinatory displacements). The obliquity of the axis of the ankle in the coronal plane causes the foot to toe out on dorsiflexion and toe in on plantar flexion.

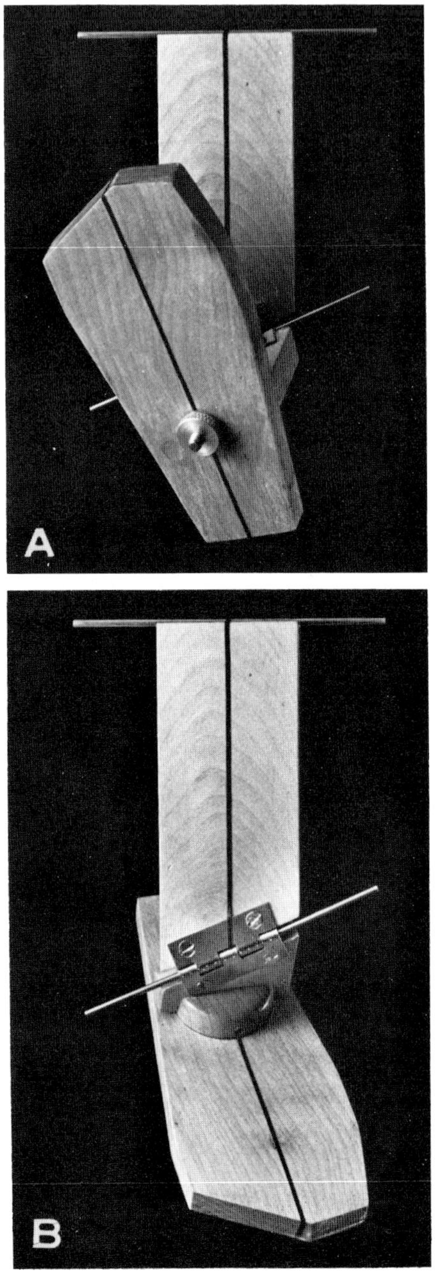

FIG. 10.7. Same arrangement of model as in Figure 10.6. For the sake of clarity the plastic disk and Devil Level have been removed and a black line has been inscribed on the vertical member to indicate the midline of the leg. Dorsiflexion to 40° is shown in *A* and plantar flexion to 40° in *B*. The toeing out on dorsiflexion and toeing in on plantar flexion, which result from the obliquity of the hinge, are clearly shown.

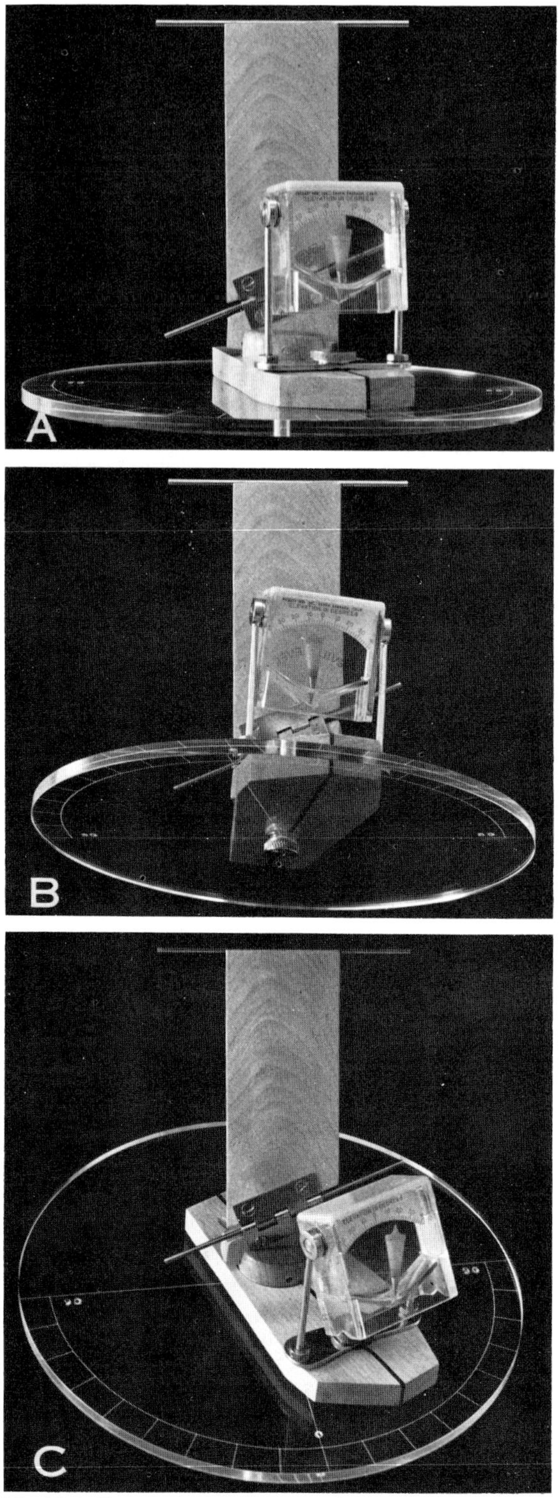

FIG. 10.8. Foot rotated medially 25° in relation to oblique axis of ankle hinge. During dorsiflexion and plantar flexion of the ankle, the vertical displacement of the foot will occur in a plane oblique by 25° to the plane of the ankle hinge. It will be seen that dorsiflexion and plantar flexion impose a longitudinal rotation of the foot as revealed by the Devil Level. Note that this longitudinal rotation is similar to that shown in Figure 10.4 and is due to the 25° of medial rotation of the foot. To this longitudinal rotation of the foot is added the toeing-in effect of the obliquely oriented ankle hinge (see Figs. 10.6 and 10.7); this is emphasized in Figure 10.7.

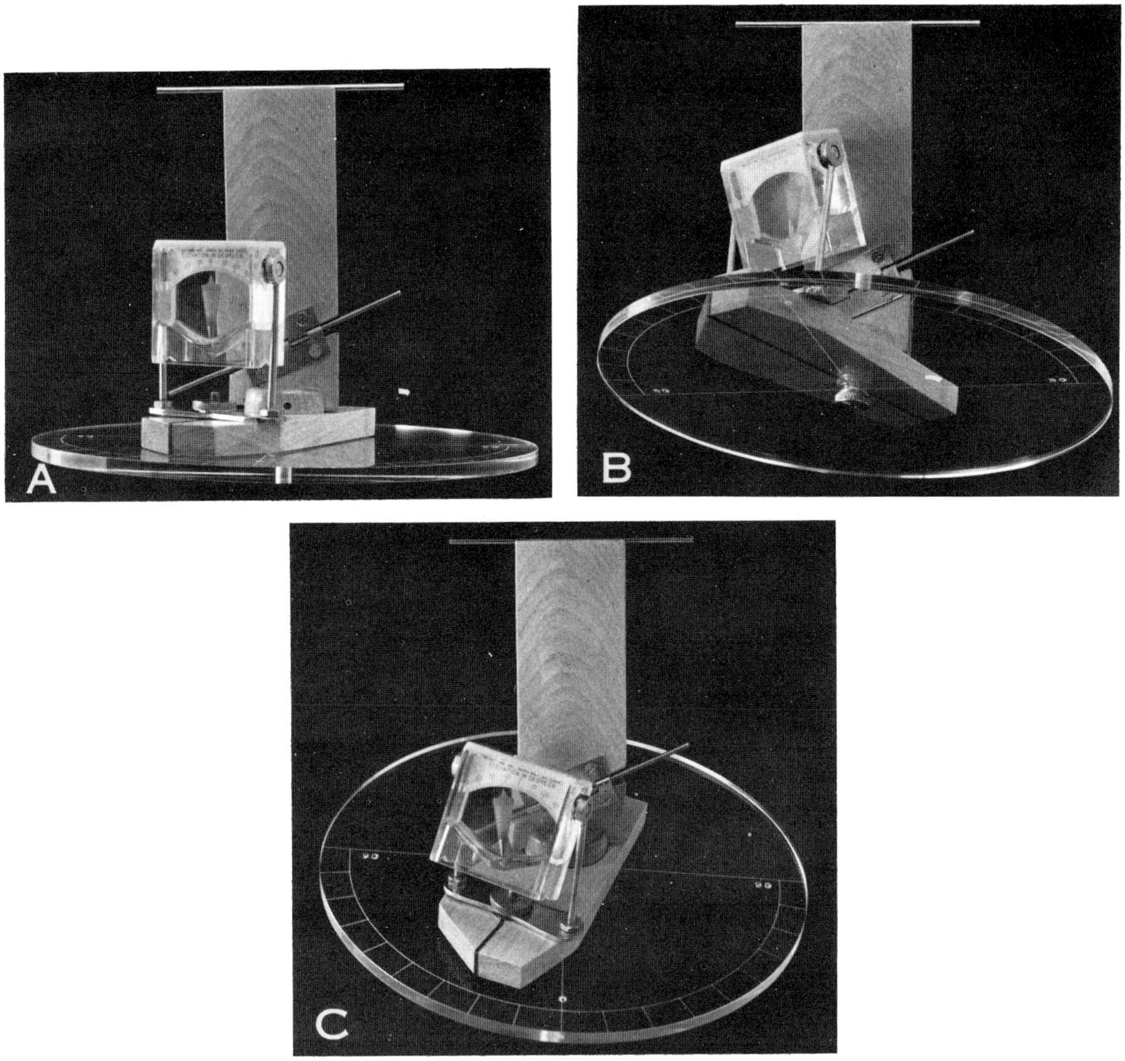

FIG. 10.9. Foot rotated laterally 25° in relation to axis of ankle joint. This orientation has caused a longitudinal rotation of the foot about its long axis, but in a reverse direction. Note that there is still a tendency for the foot to rotate medially during plantar flexion because of flexion about the obliquely oriented hinge.

FOOT FIXED, LEG FREE

Effect of an Oblique Axis of the Ankle upon the Leg with the Foot Fixed

During the stance phase of walking, when the foot is immobilized through contact with the floor, any effect of movement of the ankle about an oblique axis must be upon the leg rather than upon the foot. These effects will be presented in the following series of photographs of the wooden model. It is necessary to divide the discussion into two parts. The first part will consist of a presentation of the simple movements of dorsiflexion and plantar flexion with the various orientations of the axis. The second part will relate the effects of the changing movements of dorsiflexion and plantar flexion that occur during the stance phase of walking to certain rotatory displacements of the leg.

Effect of Varying the Axis in the Transverse Plane

Should the axis of the ankle be positioned in a horizontal plane parallel to the axis of the knee and at a right angle to the midline of the foot, the entire range of movement of the leg over the foot will obviously take place in the sagittal plane. No rotation of the leg about a vertical axis will occur (Fig. 10.10). (The same models as in Figs. 10.6 to 10.9 were used in Figs. 10.10 to 10.14, but the Devil Level and plastic disk have been removed and the model is viewed from above.)

If the axis of the ankle is medially or laterally rotated in relation to the fixed foot, then a new plane of movement is established which deviates either medially or laterally from the sagittal plane. In Figure 10.11, the axis of the ankle, while remaining horizon-

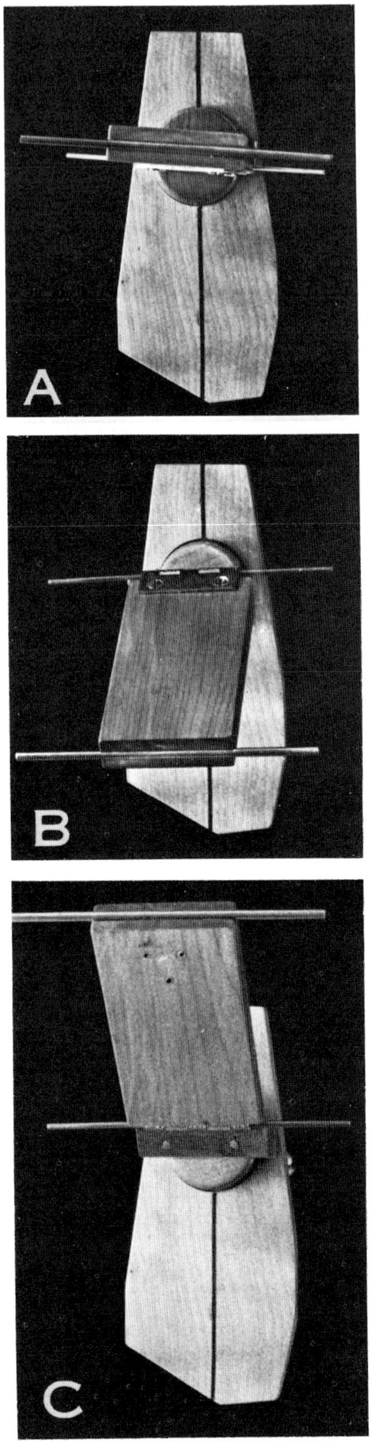

FIG. 10.10. Wooden model seen from above. The foot is fixed and the leg is moved from a neutral position (*A*) to dorsiflexion of 20° (*B*) and to plantar flexion of 30° (*C*). Note that the pins indicating the knee and ankle axes remain parallel. Movement occurs in the sagittal plane. There is no rotation of the leg about its vertical axis.

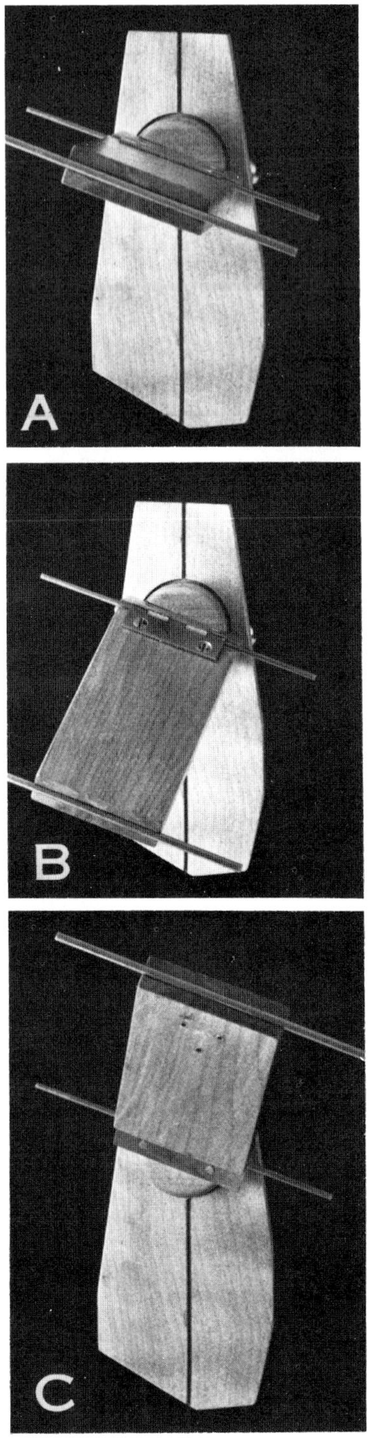

FIG. 10.11. Model with axes of knee and ankle laterally rotated in relation to midline of foot. Note that the leg again shows no rotation about a vertical axis. This is evident from the parallelism that persists between the pins that locate the knee and ankle axes. The leg moves in a plane that is oblique to the sagittal plane. This causes the leg to deviate laterally on dorsiflexion (*B*) and medially on plantar flexion (*C*).

tal, is laterally rotated in relation to the midline of the foot. The movement of the leg in the plane dictated by the new position of the axis and in a plane oblique to the sagittal plane, results in a need for the leg to incline laterally on dorsiflexion and medially on plantar flexion.

Effect of an Oblique Axis in the Coronal Plane

The anthropometric studies have demonstrated that the axis of the ankle in the coronal plane is always inclined laterally and downward to a varying amount. The effect of such an obliquely oriented axis upon the leg when it is moved over a fixed foot is shown in Figure 10.12. Movement of the leg over the fixed foot produces medial rotation of the leg on dorsiflexion and lateral rotation of the leg on plantar flexion, with little tendency for lateral or medial deviation of the leg from the sagittal plane.

That horizontal rotation of the leg about its long axis on dorsiflexion and plantar flexion actually does occur is demonstrated in an arbitrarily selected cadaver specimen (Figs. 10.13 and 10.14).

The Oblique Axis Related to Certain Clinical Observations

In review, it is hoped that the use of the wooden models has made understandable the effects of different orientations of the axis of the ankle joint.

It should be emphasized at this point that the effects reported here only grossly simulate what occurs in the living foot since in using a model of a rigid foot all other articulations in the foot that may modify the displacements of the skeletal structures located more distally are ignored. However, with this limited information, certain common observations of the behavior of the foot become explicable. These are mentioned here only to encourage others to confirm them and to seek more specific quantitative relationships.

When a person sits with thighs crossed, the relaxed free foot falls into slight plantar flexion and in so doing tends to deviate medially and to supinate slightly. This would be the natural result of an obliquely oriented ankle axis (see Figs. 10.6 and 10.7) if the subtalar joint remains in a neutral position. If the foot is gently dorsiflexed it tends to deviate laterally. Again this is what one would expect if the foot moves about an oblique axis (Figs. 10.6 and 10.7).

Inspection of the sole of the shoe reveals a worn area on the posterolateral side of the heel in most persons. It seems reasonable to link the tendency for the shoe to strike this area of the heel to the obliquity of the

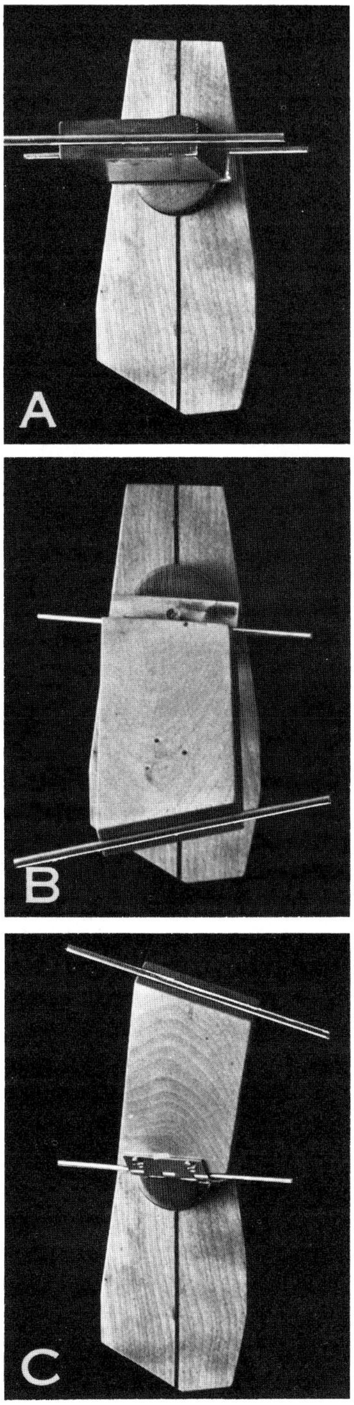

FIG. 10.12. Ankle hinge oriented obliquely in coronal plane. The orientation is the same as in Figures 10.6 to 10.9. The pins representing the knee and ankle axes are at a right angle to the midline of the foot. The effect of the oblique hinge causes a rotation of the leg about a vertical axis during movement of the leg over the fixed foot. From the neutral position (*A*), where the axes of the knee and ankle are parallel, note that on dorsiflexion (*B*) the leg rotates medially relative to the foot. On plantar flexion (*C*) the leg rotates laterally relative to the foot.

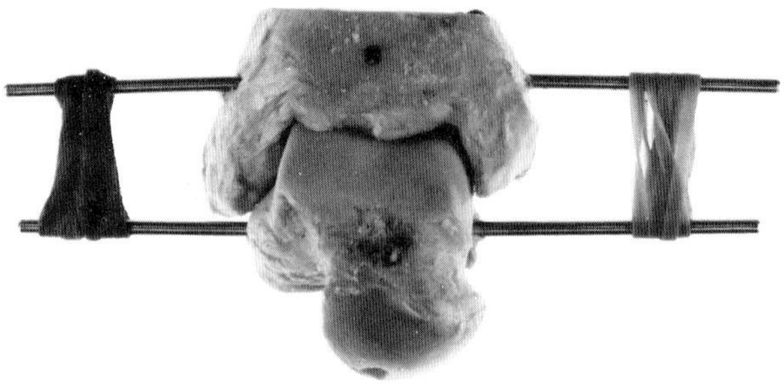

FIG. 10.13. Anatomic preparation demonstrating that an oblique axis of ankle joint causes horizontal rotation about a vertical axis between talus and leg when ankle is dorsiflexed and plantar flexed. A randomly selected specimen was used. The tibia and fibula have been cut just proximal to the ankle mortise and articulated within the talus. The articular surfaces of the ankle are held in firm apposition with rubber bands as shown in the photograph. The talus was securely fixed by a 6.4-mm bolt passed through its neck and attached to a metal base, leaving the tibia and fibula free to move.

ankle axis as it affects both leg and foot. An interesting relationship exists between the rotatory effect upon the foot resulting from different orientations of the foot in the transverse plane (refer to Figs. 10.4 and 10.5) and the deviations from the sagittal plane on movements of dorsiflexion and plantar flexion of the ankle due to the inclination of the axis in the coronal plane (refer to Fig. 10.7). This relationship is clearly demonstrated in Figures 10.8 and 10.9. It should be noted that if the foot is rotated medially, on slight dorsiflexion the heel will strike the ground relatively straight across the back. However, if the foot is rotated laterally (Fig. 10.9*B*) the heel must contact the ground more on its lateral side. There are, therefore, two variables that may affect the position of the heel at the time of heel strike. It would prove interesting to try to relate quantitatively the different positions of the worn area on the heels of the shoes of

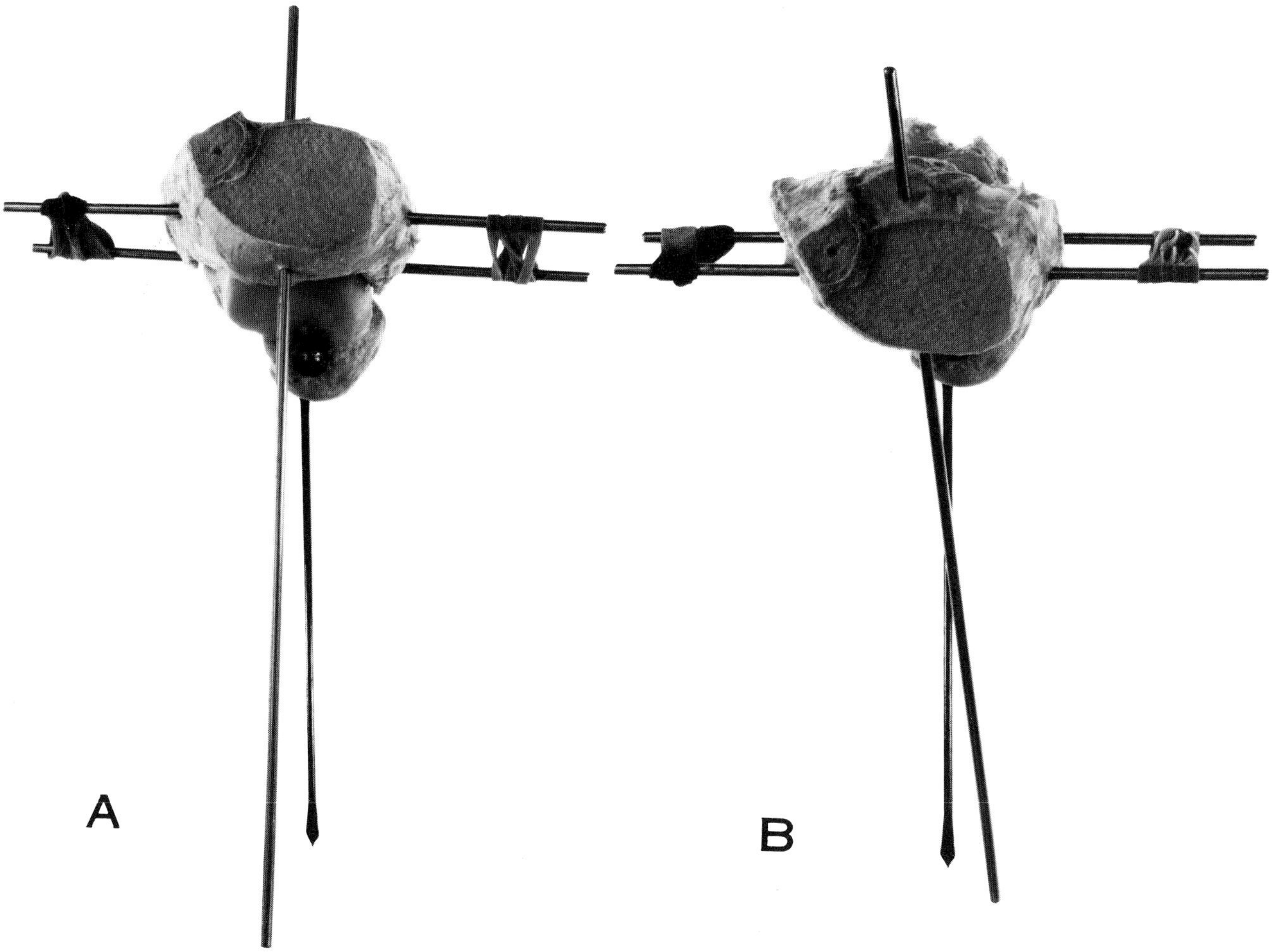

FIG. 10.14. Top view of preparation shown in Figure 10.13. Metal rods have been inserted into the talar head and the tibia to act as pointers. In *A* the ankle is in plantar flexion. Note that the two pointers diverge. In *B* the ankle is in full dorsiflexion. Note that horizontal rotation of the tibia on the talus has occurred, with crossing of the pointers.

different individuals to the varying positions of the ankle axis.

In some people the tendency of the foot to rotate medially during the short interval between heel strike and foot flat is very obvious. During this phase the foot is plantar flexing and an oblique axis of the ankle would produce just such an effect on the foot. Obviously, the degree to which this occurs would be related to the precise position of the axis and the amount of plantar flexion in the ankle occurring at this time. Again it becomes obvious that quantitative data are required to substantiate these possible relationships.

It is common knowledge that some flat feet appear to improve with the wearing of higher heels. Plantar flexion about an oblique ankle axis has been demonstrated to produce slight supination and inward displacement of the foot. Such a displacement would improve the appearance of flatfoot. The degree of improvement will obviously depend upon the degree of obliquity of the axis of the ankle. Wyller (1963) has pointed out that in those individuals who have been subjected to a subtalar arthrodesis but in whom the heel still remains in too much valgus, the appearance of the foot will be improved by placing a higher heel on the shoe. The improvement in these cases must be due primarily to the presence of an oblique axis of the ankle, since the major articulations in the hindfoot and midfoot have been immobilized by the arthrodesis. Again, the amount of improvement will depend upon the degree of obliquity of the axis of the ankle.

APPLICATIONS TO HUMAN LOCOMOTION

Certain movements of the leg and foot which occur during walking may be partially explained when one considers the oblique orientation of the axis of the ankle. During the swing phase the foot is free to move in space. From a position of approximately 30° of plantar flexion at the time of toe-off, the foot dorsiflexes for toe clearance. The vertical plane in which this motion occurs will depend upon the difference in orientation between the knee and ankle axes (tibial torsion) (see Figs. 10.2 and 10.3). The amount of rotation of the foot about its long axis will depend upon the obliquity of the ankle axis to the long axis of the foot (see Figs. 10.4 and 10.5). The inclination of the axis in the coronal plane causes the foot to deviate outward (see Figs. 10.6 and 10.7). Observation of various individuals while walking will reveal differences in the behavior of the feet during this phase of gait. The degree of toe-out or toe-in is apparent. If one observes closely, a varying degree of pronation of the foot will also be detected.

THE ANKLE DURING THE STANCE PHASE OF LOCOMOTION

The ankle joint appears to contribute more to the smooth functioning of the lower extremity during locomotion than mere dorsiflexion and plantar flexion in a sagittal plane. To properly comprehend its function requires that one visualize several rotatory displacements that occur simultaneously in the leg and foot. This may be difficult but an attempt will be made to meliorate this difficulty by limiting the discussion to the stance phase of walking and dividing the stance phase into three intervals. The first interval extends from the moment of heel strike to foot flat. The second interval is between foot flat and the instant at which the heel starts to rise. The third interval is from the beginning of heel rise to toe-off. During each interval the relationships between certain movements of the leg in space and the behavior of the ankle will be discussed.

First Interval

At this time the entire lower extremity rotates medially (Levens *et al.*, 1948). The foot participates in this rotation, but, in addition, at the instant the heel contacts the floor, the foot begins to plantar flex from its position of slight dorsiflexion. The foot has not yet been immobilized by contact with the floor and is still free to move in space. During this interval and depending upon the obliquity of the ankle axis, the foot will toe in to a varying degree (see above).

Second Interval

During this interval the foot is flat on the floor and becomes the fixed element in the lower extremity. As the leg passes over the weight-bearing foot, motion in the ankle joint becomes one of relative dorsiflexion. Reference to Figure 10.12 reveals that such a movement causes a medial rotation of the leg about a vertical axis. This is precisely what occurs in the leg during this interval; *i.e.*, it continues to rotate medially (Berry, 1952).

Third Interval

As the heel starts to rise, the motion of the ankle becomes one of relative plantar flexion. If Figure 10.12 is again referred to, it will be seen that plantar flexion

(Fig. 10.12*C*) causes the leg to rotate laterally. Independent observations on the longitudinal rotations of the leg reveal that there occurs at this time an abrupt change from medial rotation of the leg to one of lateral rotation, which continues until toe-off.

In summary, the oblique ankle axis produces the following series of events. From the instant of heel contact to the time the foot is flat, plantar flexion occurs and the foot appears to toe in. The more oblique the axis, the more apparent the toeing in. During midstance, the foot is fixed on the ground; relative dorsiflexion, with resulting medial rotation of the leg, occurs as the leg passes over the foot. As the heel rises, plantar flexion takes place which results in lateral rotation of the leg.

Rotation of the leg and movements of the foot caused by an oblique ankle axis, when observed independently, are seen to be qualitatively and temporally in agreement. However, when the magnitudes of the various displacements are studied, irreconcilable disparities are evident. In normal locomotion ankle motion ranges from 20 to 36°, with an average of 24° (Ryker, 1952; Berry, 1952). The obliquity of the ankle axis ranges from 2 to 23°, with an average of 12° from the horizontal (Isman and Inman, 1968). Even in the most oblique axis and movement of the ankle through the maximal range of 36°, only 11° of rotation of the leg around a vertical axis will occur. This is less than the average amount of horizontal rotation of the leg as measured independently in normal walking. The average obliquity of the ankle, together with the average amount of dorsiflexion and plantar flexion, would yield values for the horizontal rotation of the leg which are much smaller than the degree of horizontal rotation of the leg that actually occurs while the foot remains stationary on the floor and is carrying the superincumbent body weight.

It appears from the foregoing discussion that the horizontal rotations of the leg require the participation of articulations more distally placed in the foot. The subtalar joint appears to be admirably designed to perform this task. Again, the close interrelationship between the functions of the ankle and subtalar joints becomes evident and will be discussed in detail in Chapter 12.

11

Biomechanics of the Subtalar Joint

To demonstrate the effect of the variations in the orientation of the axis of the subtalar joint, wooden models will again be used. For maximal simplicity, all other joints are ignored. The foot is represented as a rigid member and the leg as a vertical piece of wood. The only connection between the foot and the leg is a simple hinge whose orientation will be varied.

LEG FIXED, FOOT FREE

In the first series of photographs, the leg remains fixed in space and the foot moves around the axis of a hinge. The hinge remains in the sagittal plane of the leg and the midline of the foot. However, the inclination of the hinge in the vertical plane will be varied in the first series of photographs. Three positions of the hinge are depicted. Two are extreme and exceed any possible anatomic relationship of the parts; they are presented to emphasize certain relationships (Figs. 11.1 and 11.2). An intermediate position is shown which more nearly represents the average position of the axis of the subtalar joint (Fig. 11.3).

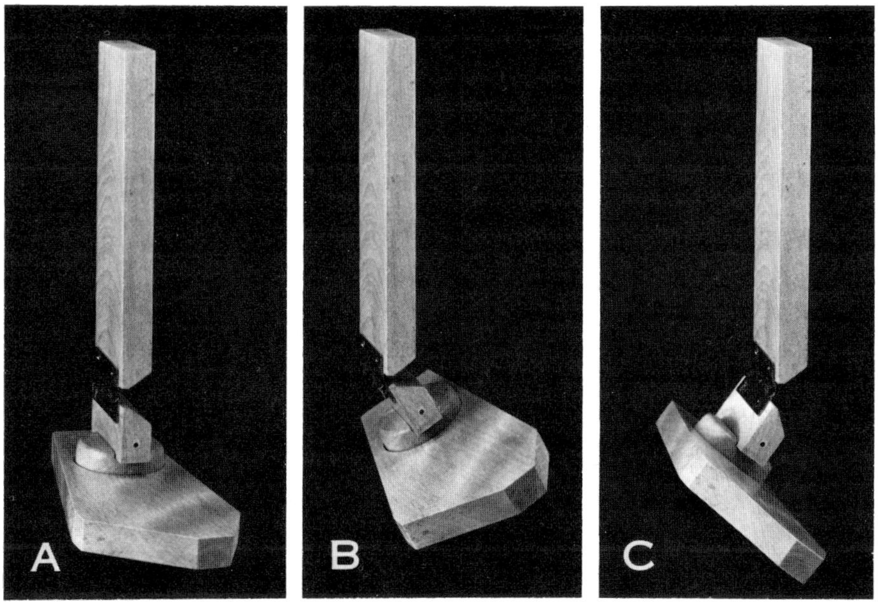

FIG. 11.1. Horizontal orientation of axis of subtalar joint (*A*). Note that a horizontal axis permits only inversion (*B*) and eversion (*C*) of the foot.

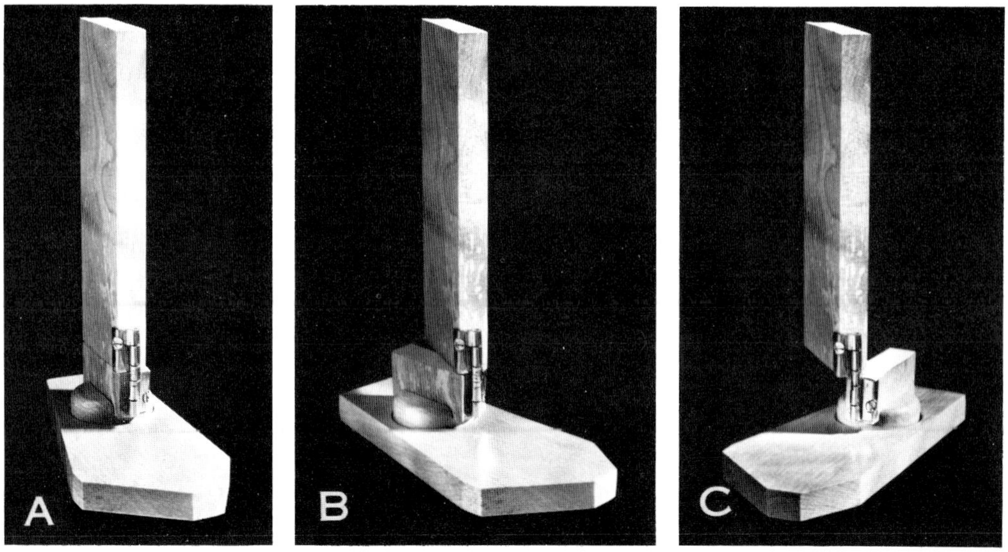

FIG. 11.2. Vertical orientation of axis of subtalar joint. Note that movement about a vertical axis causes the foot, starting from a neutral position (*A*) to adduct (toe in) (*B*), or to abduct (toe out) (*C*) in the horizontal plane. There is no accompanying eversion or inversion of the foot.

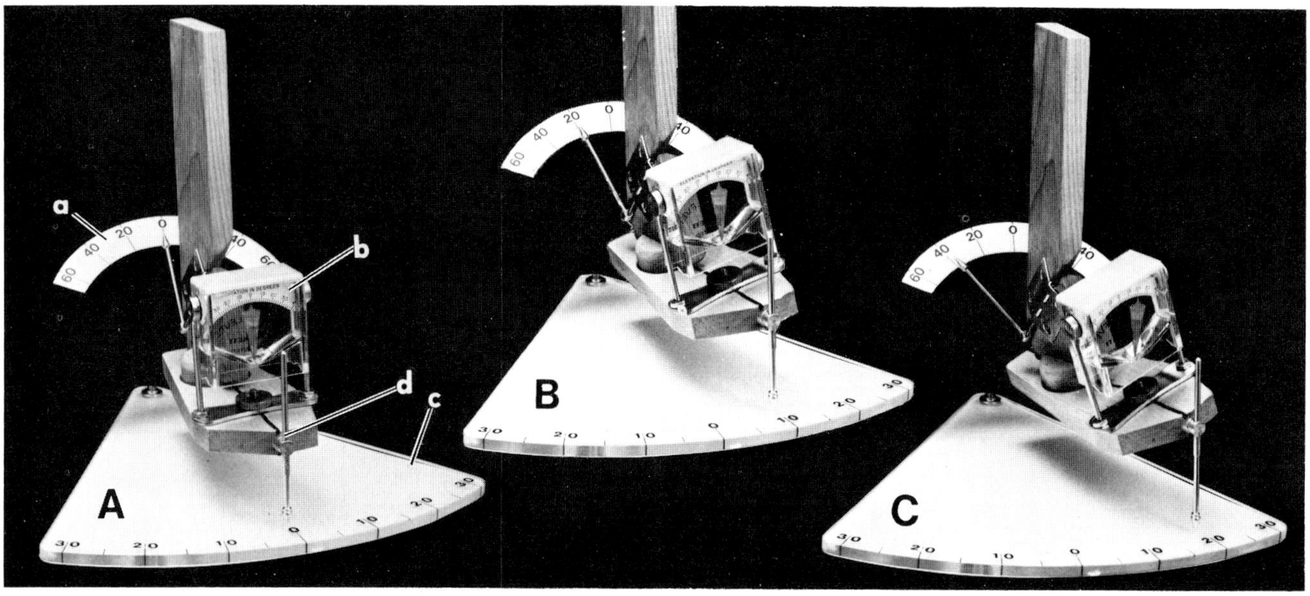

FIG. 11.3. Subtalar axis inclined to approximate average orientation. In these photographs the hinge connecting the leg and the foot of the model is inclined at 45°(midway between the horizontal, as shown in Fig. 11.1, and the vertical, as shown in Fig. 11.2). Various devices have been added to record angular changes in three planes of space: a goniometer (*a*) indicating actual amount of rotation that occurs in hinge; a Devil Level (*b*) mounted on foot to indicate amount that foot rotates (inverts) about its long axis; a horizontal scale (*c*), supported independently, has been placed below the model; a pendulum pointer (*d*) has been attached to the foot. The scale and pointer together constitute a goniometer that records the amount of adduction (toe-in) that occurs with movement of the subtalar joint. *A*, Neutral position. *B*, Subtalar joint rotated 20°. *C*, Subtalar joint rotated 40° in same direction. Note that a 45° inclination of the axis results in the total amount of movement in the subtalar joint being divided equally between rotation of the foot about its long axis (inversion) and adduction (toe-in). While only inversion and adduction are shown in these photographs, it should be apparent that the same relationships will obtain when the opposite rotation of the subtalar joint (hinge) occurs.

The following deductions should be obvious. If the subtalar axis were horizontal (parallel to the plantar surface of the foot and at an angle of 90° to the leg) movement of the foot would be one of pure rotation around a horizontal axis with the foot inverting or everting. At the other extreme, should the axis be vertical (parallel to the leg and at an angle of 90° to the foot) movement of the foot would be one of pure adduction (toeing in) or abduction (toeing out) of the forefoot. The subtalar axis, however, lies between these extremes and therefore movement of the foot will necessarily be some combination of both of these displacements.

If the axis is located at a 45° angle between the foot and the leg, the amount of rotation (inversion and eversion) and the amount of adduction and abduction of the forefoot (toeing in and toeing out) with movement of the foot about the subtalar axis hinge will be equal.

The subtalar axis, however, is rarely oriented at exactly 45° to the horizontal (the average is 42°), and it has been shown to vary within the population between the extremes of approximately 20 and 60°. A moment's reflection and a review of Figures 11.1 to 11.3 will reveal the fact that the more horizontal the subtalar axis, the more inversion and eversion will predominate over adduction and abduction, and that the more vertical the axis, the more adduction and abduction will predominate over inversion and eversion. This is pictorially demonstrated in Figures 11.4 and 11.5, where the axis of the subtalar joint has been oriented at 30° (Fig. 11.4) and 60° (Fig. 11.5) to the horizontal plane. For those who are mathematically inclined it should be apparent that the relationship between adduction-abduction and inversion-eversion varies as the tangent of the angle of inclination of the axis of the subtalar joint.

The situation described above is somewhat oversimplified, for in reality the axis of the subtalar joint does not normally lie in the same vertical plane as the leg and the midline of the foot. Posteriorly it inclines laterally as well as downward. When measured in a horizontal plane from the midline of the foot, the variation in position may be from 4 to 47°. This adds a complicating factor to the description given above and requires further discussion. However, since the horizontal deviation has been shown to be always in one direction, i.e., with the axis running posteriorly and laterally, this is the only situation that need be considered. Even so we are now dealing with two independent variables and the description becomes rather complicated. To simplify the presentation the vertical inclination of the axis will remain fixed at 45° and the effect of the lateral orientation of the axis of the subtalar joint will be presented in only a qualitative manner. Reference to Figure 11.6 should make it clear that the more the subtalar axis diverges laterally from the midline of the foot, the more it will approximate the function of an ankle joint. To the rotation (inversion and eversion) of the foot about its midline and adduction (toeing in) and abduction (toeing out) is now added a varying amount of plantar flexion and dorsiflexion.

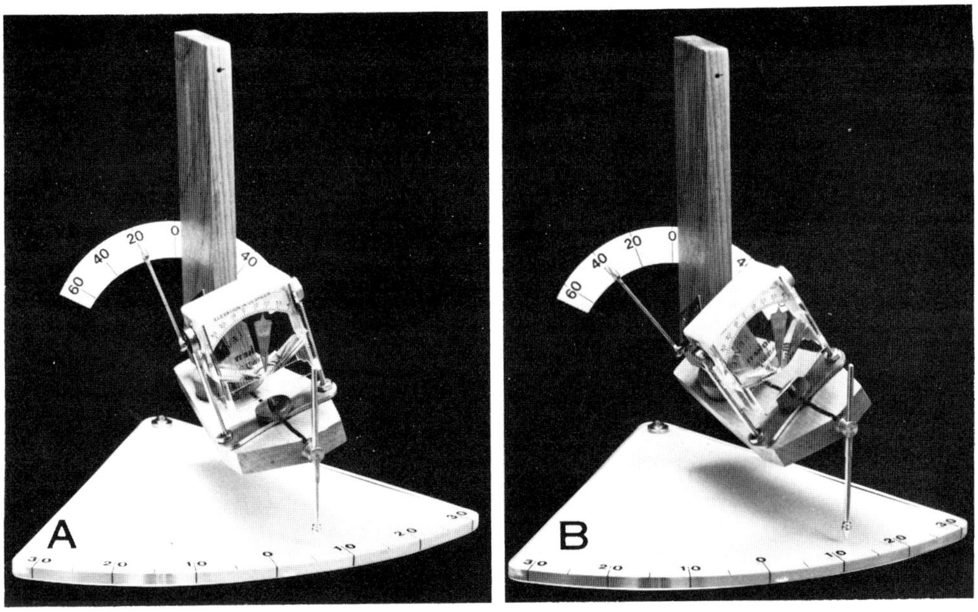

FIG. 11.4. Subtalar axis inclined 30° to horizontal. Note the more horizontal orientation of the axis than in Figure 11.3, resulting in increased inversion and decreased adduction of the foot. In *A*, 20° of rotation has occurred in the subtalar joint and in *B*, 40° of rotation is shown. Comparisons between the amounts of inversion and adduction may be made by reading the angular values from the Devil Level and the horizontal goniometer.

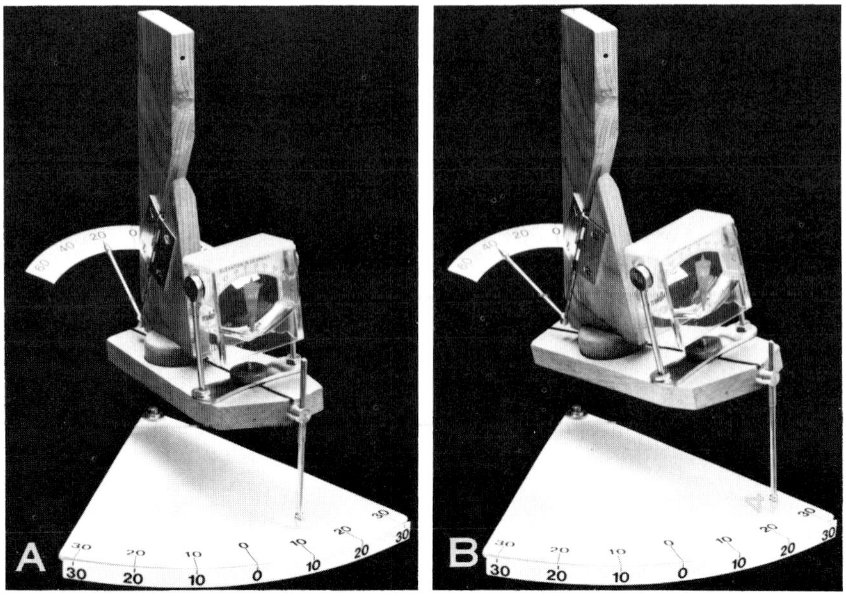

FIG. 11.5 Subtalar axis inclined 60° to horizontal. Note that the more vertically oriented axis results in suppression of inversion and an increase in the amount of adduction of the foot with the same degree of rotation of the subtalar joint. Values from the Devil Level and horizontal goniometer can be compared as the subtalar joint is rotated 20° in *A* and 40° in *B*.

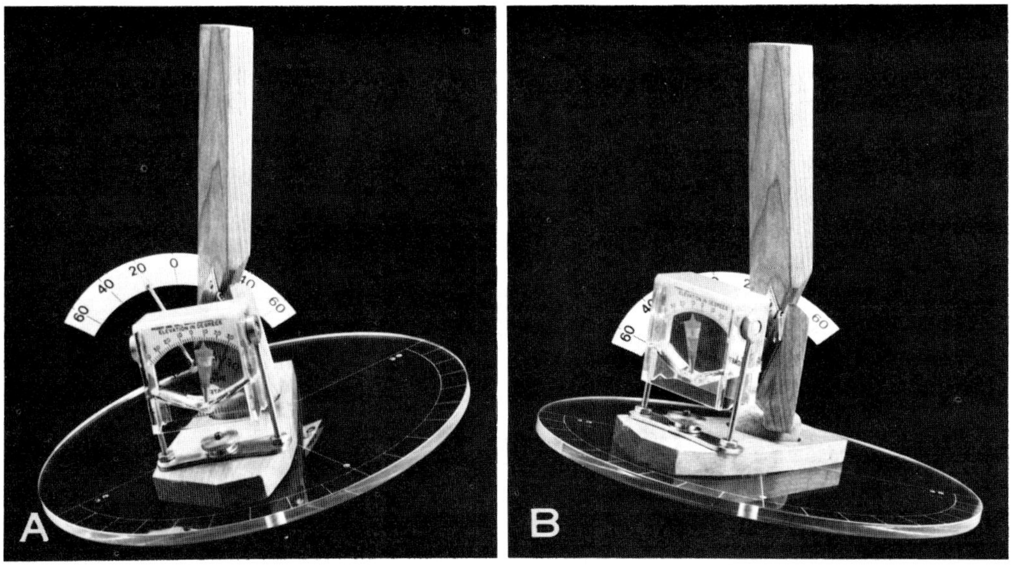

FIG. 11.6. Effect of posterolateral deviation of axis of subtalar joint from midline of foot. To depict the factor of plantar flexion and dorsiflexion in addition to the previously demonstrated inversion-eversion and adduction-abduction displacements (see Figs. 11.1 to 11.3), a circular plastic disk has been attached to the foot of the model. The disk has been inscribed in 10° increments, from 0 to 90°. The 0° diameter remains parallel to the anteroposterior plane of the hinge, while the diameters connecting the 90° inscriptions remain perpendicular to the plane of the hinge. The degree of posterolateral deviation of the subtalar joint (hinge) from the midline of the foot can be read from the inscriptions on the disk. Two views only are presented in this figure. In both photographs the foot has been rotated outward so that the axis of the subtalar joint makes an angle of 40° with the midline of the foot. Note that in *A*, motion of 20° in the subtalar joint causes the foot to invert and adduct as previously demonstrated but also imposes a degree of plantar flexion. In *B* the reverse displacements are shown.

FOOT FIXED, LEG FREE

When the foot is immobilized, movement in the subtalar joint can occur only through lateral or medial deviation of the leg upon the foot. Because of the obliquity of the subtalar axis the medial and lateral displacements of the leg are accompanied by rotations of the leg in a transverse plane (about a longitudinal axis). This is shown in Figure 11.7, in which the subtalar axis is inclined 45°. A moment of reflection should make it apparent to the reader that the relationship between the medial and lateral displacements of the leg and the extent of transverse rotation of the leg are related to the inclination of the subtalar axis. A more horizontal position of the subtalar axis will cause less transverse rotation, while a more vertical axis will impose a greater amount of rotation with the same amount of motion in the subtalar joint.

The usual activities of daily living rarely demand lateral and medial deviations of the leg upon a fixed foot. During ambulation, the tibia remains in a relatively vertical plane during the stance phase. In athletic competition, however, deviations of the leg from the vertical are a common occurrence. One need only review the action photographs published in a sports magazine to see marked inclinations of the leg upon a fixed foot. This would be impossible without a subtalar joint (Figs. 11.8 and 11.9).

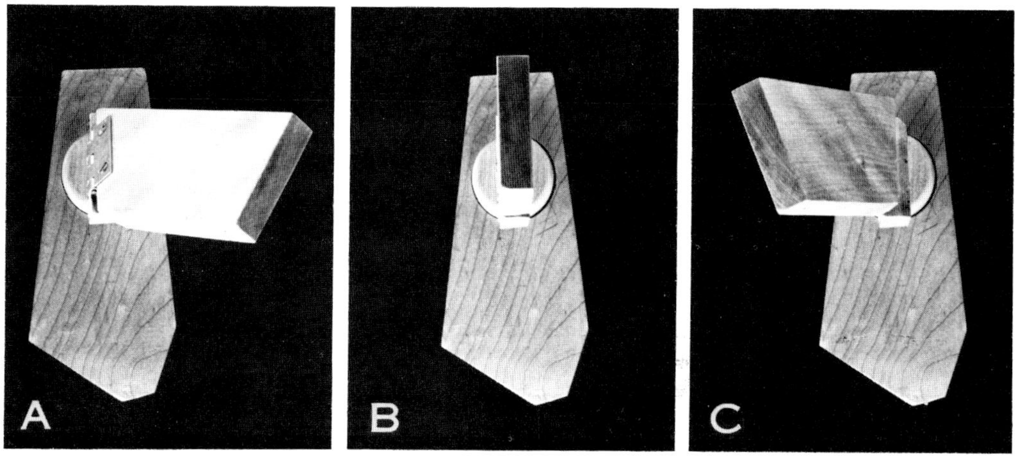

FIG. 11.7. Movement of subtalar joint with foot immobilized. The model demonstrates clearly that with a fixed foot, motion in the subtalar joint can only occur through lateral or medial deviation of the leg. In these photographs the subtalar axis is inclined 45°. This inclination imposes longitudinal rotations of the leg which must accompany the lateral and medial deviations.

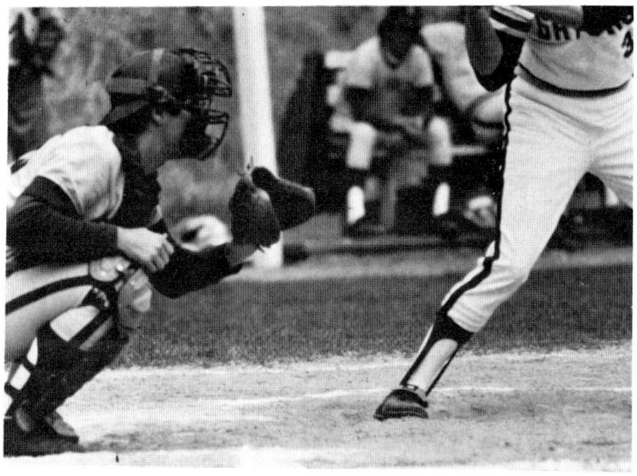

FIG. 11.8. Baseball action photograph showing motion at subtalar joint. Note the position of the right leg of the man at bat. The leg is inclined approximately 35° from the vertical plane, while the foot remains relatively flat on the ground. However, the leg has been internally rotated; this rotation, through the action of the subtalar joint (see Figs. 9.3, 11.13, and 11.14), has caused the foot to pronate, thus driving the medial side of the shoe into the ground.

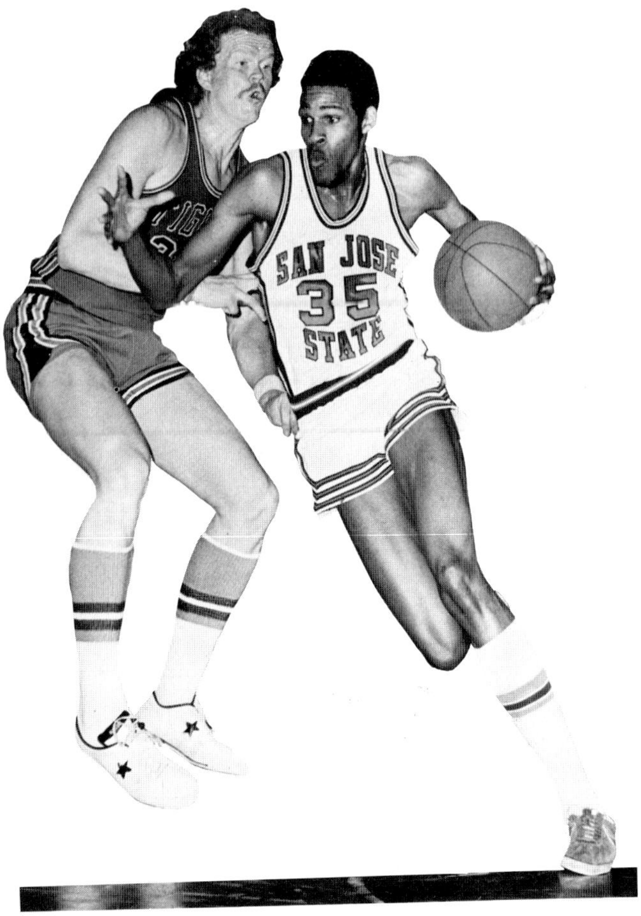

FIG. 11.9. Subtalar motion. Note the position of the left leg and foot of the basketball player as he drives in under the basket. Approximately 45° of motion has occurred in the subtalar joint. (Courtesy of the San Jose Mercury Herald)

THE SUBTALAR JOINT—A DIRECTIONAL TORQUE TRANSMITTER

The importance of the subtalar joint in permitting transverse rotation of the leg to occur during the stance phase of walking has been mentioned briefly in a previous section. A more detailed discussion is presented at this time.

One should recall that human walking is more than merely the oscillation of two legs in the plane of progression. There occurs a series of rotations in which all segments participate. The pelvis rotates in a horizontal plane around the weight-bearing hip. The total amount of this rotation varies from individual to individual about a mean of approximately 8° (Saunders *et al.*, 1953). The thigh rotates in phase with the pelvic rotation, but to a greater extent, and the shank (tibia) even more. The average rotation of the shank has been found to be 19°, with a range of 13 to 26° (Levens *et al.*, 1948). The foot normally does not slip on the floor; thus a mechanism must exist between the lower leg (shank) and the floor which permits these rotations to occur. While mention has been made that a very oblique ankle joint may subserve this function to a limited extent, the main responsibility resides in the subtalar joint.

Wooden models will again be utilized to demonstrate the capability of the subtalar joint to allow the leg to rotate medially and laterally while remaining vertical and without the foot adducting or abducting through slippage on the floor. Particular attention should be called, however, to the inversion (supination) and eversion (pronation) of the foot which necessarily accompany the rotations of the leg. The rotations of the leg about a vertical axis are converted into rotations of the foot about a horizontal axis.

In Figures 11.10 and 11.11 the axis of the subtalar joint is oriented parallel to the midline of the foot and inclined at 45° to the horizontal. The model demonstrates that with a 45° inclination of the subtalar axis, medial and lateral rotation of the leg causes equal amounts of eversion (pronation) and inversion (supination) of the foot.

Attention is again called to the fact that the average inclination of the subtalar axis is less than 45° (average 42°), and wide individual variations from this average occur within the population. The effects of a more horizontal or a more vertical orientation of the axis are shown in Figures 11.12 and 11.13.

The functional relationship between medial-lateral rotation of the leg and pronation-supination of the foot due to the presence of a subtalar joint is readily demonstrated in any normal person. In Figure 11.14 pointers have been attached to the leg and foot to assist in the visualization of these rotations.

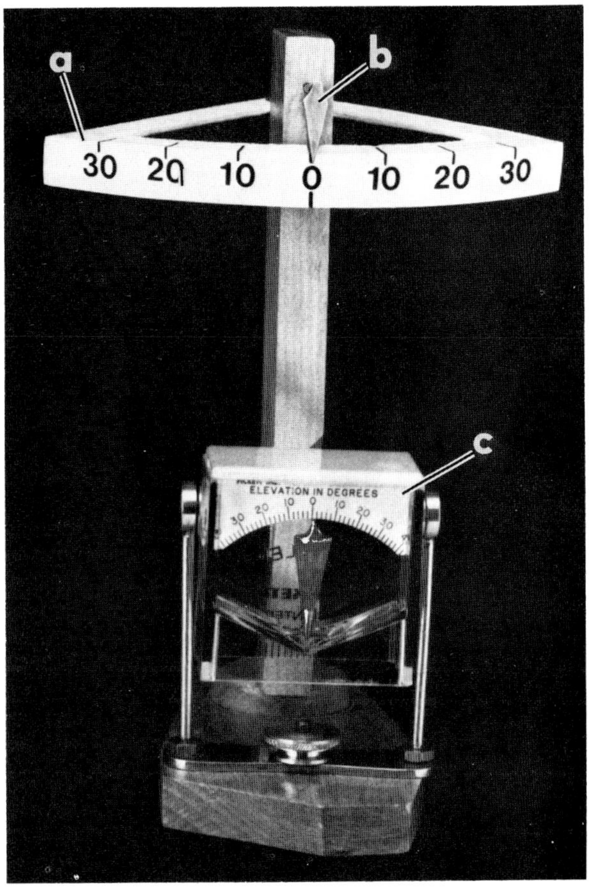

FIG. 11.10. Subtalar joint as directional torque transmitter. The wooden model selected has the subtalar axis oriented at 45° to the horizontal and in line with the midline of the foot. It is mounted so that the vertical member representing the leg remains vertical but can be rotated in a transverse plane about its long axis. A scale (*a*) is supported independently of the model. A pointer (*b*) is attached to the vertical member; *a* and *b* constitute a goniometer that records the amount of internal and external rotation of the leg. The foot will remain in the sagittal plane but can rotate about a horizontal axis (pronate or supinate). The degree of pronation or supination is recorded by the Devil Level (*c*). The relationship of internal and external rotation of the leg to pronation and supination of the foot is revealed in the following series of photographs (Fig. 11.11).

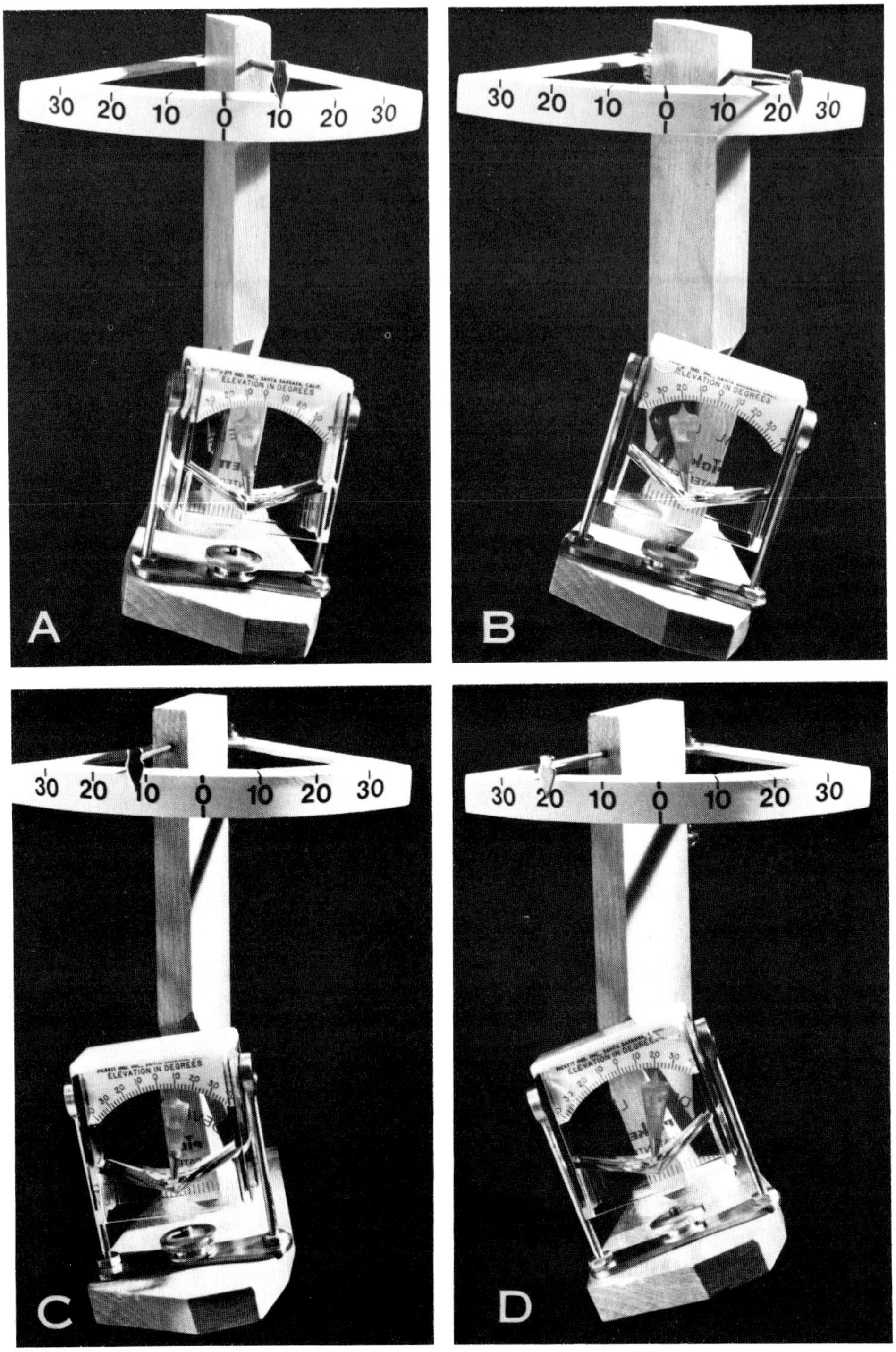

FIG. 11.11. Relationship between rotation of leg and pronation-supination of foot. Medial rotation of the leg is shown in *A* and *B*. Note that the foot pronates an equal amount as indicated by the Devil Level. Lateral rotation is shown in *C* and *D*. Note that the foot supinates the same amount. This equality in angular displacements exists only if the subtalar axis is inclined at 45°.

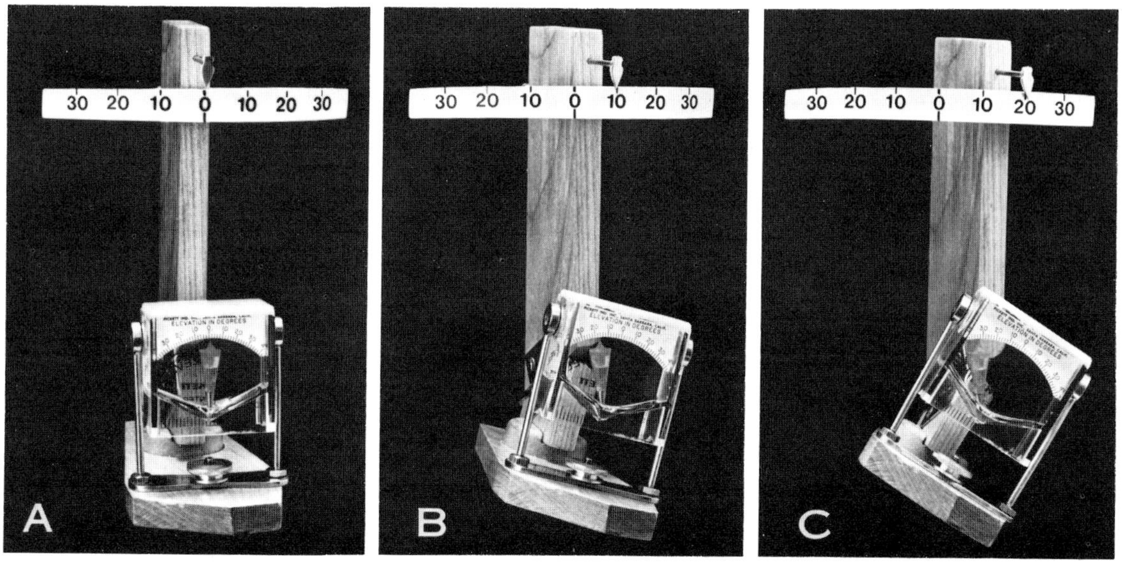

FIG. 11.12. Effect of more horizontal orientation of subtalar axis. In this series of photographs, the subtalar axis has been inclined 30° to the horizontal. Only medial rotation of the leg is shown since lateral rotation would show the same values for the displacements but in the opposite direction. Note that the same amount of internal rotation produces a greater amount of pronation of the foot, as recorded by the Devil Level.

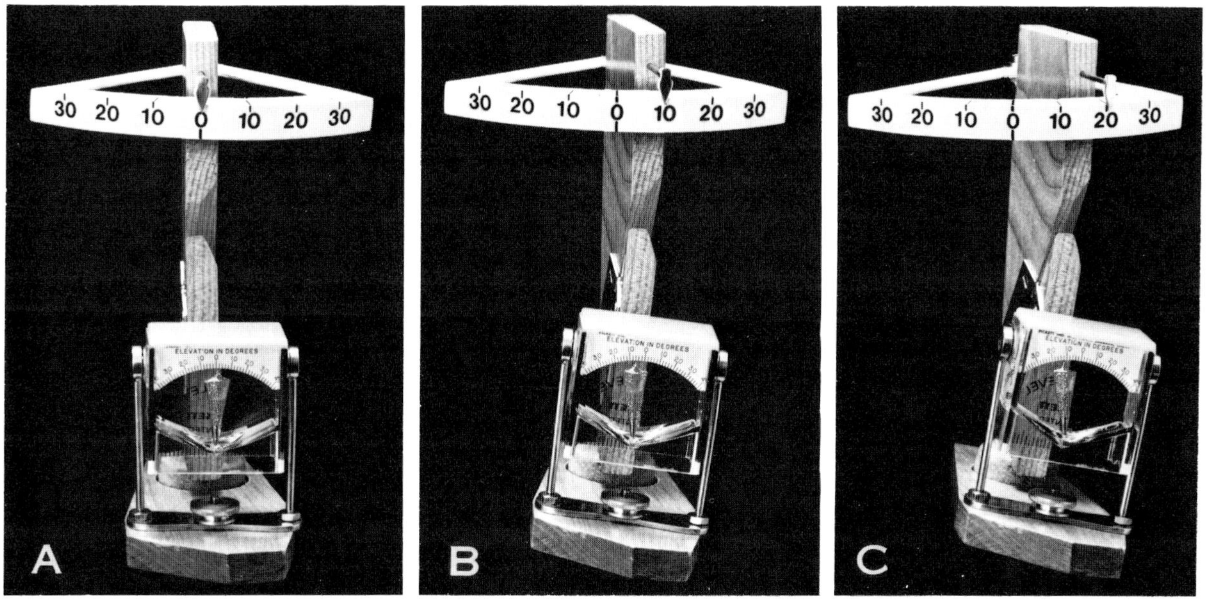

FIG. 11.13. Effect of more vertical orientation of subtalar axis. In this series the subtalar axis has been inclined 60 °to the horizontal. Note that the more vertical orientation of the axis permits medial rotation of the leg with less pronation of the foot.

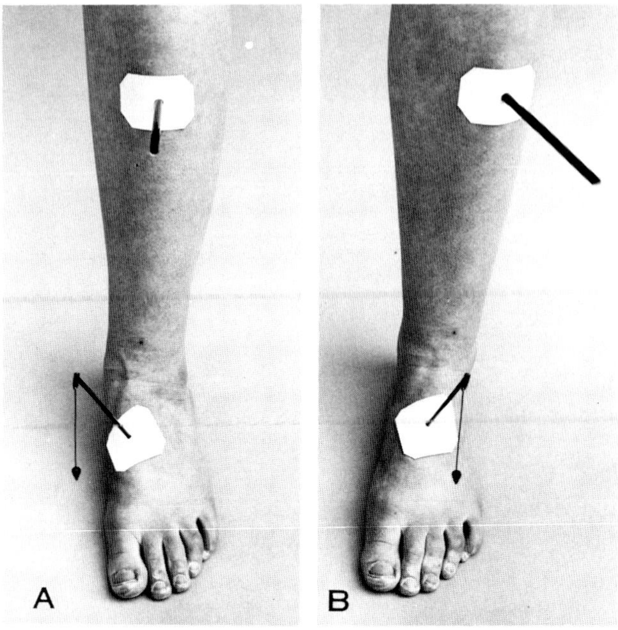

FIG. 11.14. Subtalar joint as directional torque transmitter. Pointers have been taped to the leg and foot of an arbitrarily selected subject. To provide better visualization of the amount of pronation and supination of the foot, a pendulum has been added to the pointer which has been taped to the dorsum of the foot. In *A* the leg is medially rotated with accompanying pronation of the foot. In *B* the leg is laterally rotated with supination of the foot.

12

The Ankle and Subtalar Joints in Walking

If the reader has had the patience to study the material so far presented it should have become apparent that the ankle and subtalar joints constitute an integrated mechanism and the function of one can not be studied to the exclusion of the other. Wright *et al.* (1964) have likened the two joints to the component parts of a universal coupling (a cardan joint). This concept is true only to a limited extent. In a universal coupling the two axes of motion intersect and are located perpendicular to one another. This is not true of the axes of the ankle and subtalar joints, which have been shown to vary not only in their positions relative to the leg and foot but to each other. Furthermore, while anatomically the axes may remain in a fixed position in any one person, their positions in space change with changing movements of the leg and foot. This is true in walking and is due principally to the transverse rotations that occur in the leg. These changing orientations of the axes lead to variations both in the amount of motion contributed by each joint and in their phasic relationships (the times at which these rotations occur).

Unfortunately only one study has been reported (Wright *et al.*) which recorded the simultaneous motions in both the ankle and subtalar joints during locomotion. These authors carefully studied two individuals with an instrumented mechanical analogue fixed to the leg and shoe. The unit was adjusted so that the axes of the mechanical and anatomic joints were coincident. Potentiometers were incorporated in the mechanical axes which recorded rotations about both ankle and subtalar axes individually and simultaneously. Figure 12.1 has been redrawn from this study. It illustrates the participation of each joint in normal walking and the variable effects of toeing in and toeing out on the behavior of each joint.

Figure 12.1 is a recording of the simultaneous rotations of the ankle and subtalar joints during normal walking in one subject. The stance phase of walking is divided into three intervals. The first interval extends from heel contact to foot flat. Note that during this phase the ankle plantar flexes and simultaneously the foot pronates as revealed by the angular displacement recorded by the potentiometer aligned with the axes of the joints. During the second interval, the foot remains flat and immobile on the floor while the body moves forward over the weight-bearing leg. The ankle dorsiflexes and the foot progressively supinates. The third interval starts at the instant the heel begins to rise and terminates with toe-off. This interval is characterized by rapid plantar flexion of the ankle while the foot continues to supinate. These recordings clearly demonstrate the participation of both ankle and subtalar joints in normal walking on a level surface.

In normal locomotion the angular displacement in the subtalar joint is approximately one-half as much as that in the ankle joint. However, reorienting the axes to the plane of progression by having the subject walk toeing out or toeing in leads to interesting changes in the patterns of movement in both the ankle and subtalar joints. Toeing out caused an increase in the amount of rotation in the subtalar joint and a slight decrease in the angular displacement in the ankle joint. Toeing in suppressed the supination of the foot during the entire second inter-

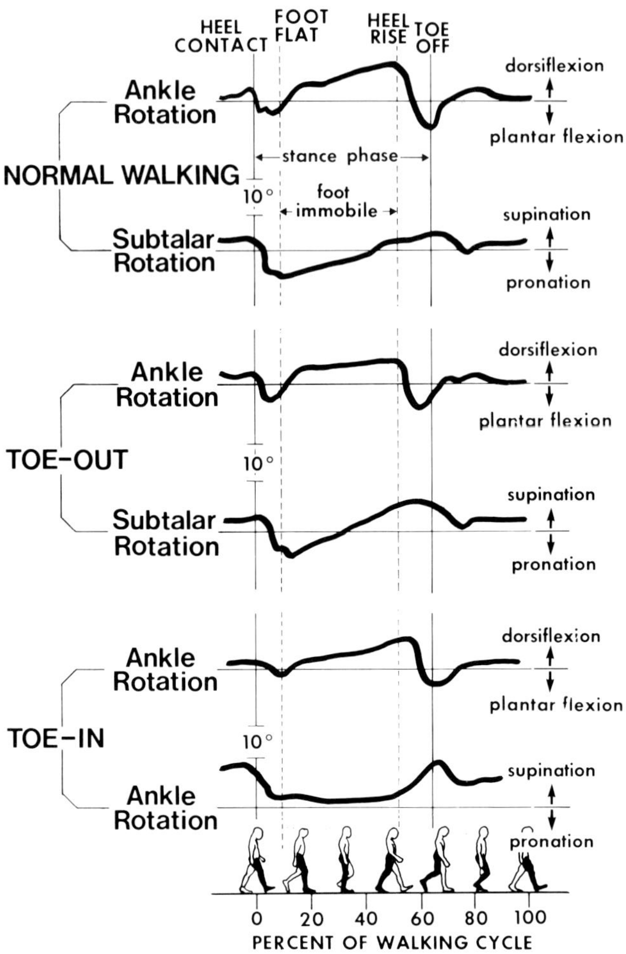

FIG. 12.1. Simultaneous rotations in ankle and subtalar joints in walking. Note the variations in the phases of motion as well as the ranges of movement with different degrees of toe-in and toe-out. (Redrawn with permission, from Wright, D. B., Desai, S. M., and Henderson, W. H. Action of the subtalar and ankle-joint complex during the stance phase of walking. *J. Bone Joint Surg.* 46A:361, 1964)

val and caused rapid and exaggerated supination during heel rise.

The two subjects studied by Wright *et al.* showed similar patterns of movement in the ankle and subtalar joints, but additional studies are needed before specific relationships can be established between ankle and subtalar motion. It appears likely that the variations in the obliquity of the ankle axis and the variations in the inclination of the subtalar axis will lead to different patterns of motion, as well as to differences in magnitude of the angular displacements in the two joints in various individuals. Such a study is necessary before any causal relationships can be established in a variety of published clinical observations, for example, between tarsal coalitions and "ball-and-socket" ankle joints, between subtalar fusions and degenerative arthritis of the ankle joint, or between ankle arthrodesis and degenerative arthritis of the tarsal joints. Furthermore, the future design and development of internal prostheses for the ankle should be based upon adequate quantitative data. These data should certainly take into consideration the presence or absence of residual subtalar motion. Several types of prostheses may be required depending upon whether subtalar motion need be supplied or not.

13

Applications to Orthopaedics and Areas for Further Clinical Research

Where clinical observations appear to be explained directly through application of the concept presented in the body of the monograph, they have been included in the text. It is therefore redundant to do more than list those items which have been previously discussed. However, there seem to be additional relationships between certain clinical observations and the newer concepts of the function of the ankle and subtalar joints which are only alluded to in the text. These will be discussed in a more extensive manner. It is hoped that the suggestion of possible correlations will encourage others to seek specific answers through further clinical research. This chapter, therefore, will consist of a brief review of assorted injuries and abnormalities of the ankle and hindfoot. The material is grouped into general categories under separate titles.

LOCOMOTION

The interrelationship between the ankle and subtalar joints in normal locomotion has been discussed in the text (pp. 67–68). The appreciation that such a relationship exists needs to be followed by the collection of adequate data on patients who have lost the function of one or the other joint through trauma or surgical procedures. These must be supplemented with a long-term follow-up.

The improvement achieved by the wearing of high heels in the appearance of pes planus and in the persistence of a valgus heel has been discussed in the test (p. 55). Note that the degree of improvement will depend upon the obliquity of the ankle axis as projected upon a coronal plane.

The effect of toeing in and toeing out in altering the degree of participation of the ankle and subtalar joints has been shown (pp. 67–68).

DEVELOPMENTAL ABNORMALITIES

"Ball-and-Socket" Ankle Joints

It is regrettable that most reports of "ball-and-socket" ankle joints in the literature have failed to record whether abnormalities were present in the foot which limited subtalar function and therefore imposed abnormally large rotatory forces on the ankle in the growing child. Furthermore, the ability of the ankle to absorb these forces depends upon its obliquity (see Figs. 10.12–10.14). As yet no data have been available as to the obliquity of the axis as estimated in the x-rays by drawing a line between the tips of the malleoli (p. 9).

Valgus and Varus Deformities

Both shortening and overgrowth of the lateral malleolus have been cited as causes for deformities of the ankle. Children with pseudarthrosis of the fibula with accompanying shortening of the lateral malleolus tend to develop an increasing valgus of the ankle. The same situation has occurred in children in whom a segment of the fibula has been removed to furnish bone for grafting (Hsu *et al.*, 1972; Wiltse, 1972), as well as in congenital shortening (Middleton, 1975). Conversely, overgrowth of the fibula has led to a varus deformity of the ankle (Makin, 1965).

Whether these deformities are the result of the loss or the existence of lateral pressures exerted by the malleolus against the trochlea, of changes in the axis of motion of the ankle, of alterations in the ligamentous support, or of changes in the percentage of body weight transmitted by the fibula (Lambert, 1971) is still an unanswered question.

ACQUIRED DISORDERS

Before one can understand the factors involved in the disorders to be discussed presently, it is necessary to review some aspects of the anatomy of the ligaments and expand on their functional behavior during movement of the ankle joint.

The descriptive anatomy of the lateral collateral ligaments has been discussed in some detail in the text (pp. 30–34). Special attention was called to the calcaneofibular ligament, about which two facts were presented at that time. First, this ligament is constant; it has been reported to be present as a distinct and strong structure in all primate and prosimian species. In all probability it is present in other mammalian species as well, but reports in the literature are lacking. Second, it passes over two joints, *i.e.*, the talocrural and talocalcaneal joints, and therefore must be examined in the light of both ankle and subtalar motion. Now that adequate anthropometric data on these two joints have been presented, it is possible to examine critically the anatomic arrangement and functional characteristics of the calcaneofibular ligament.

The necessity for the ligament to pursue an oblique course downward and backward from the fibula to the calcaneus will be demonstrated and in the course of this demonstration an explanation for several reported clinical observations will become evident.

Since the calcaneofibular ligament passes over both the ankle and the subtalar joints it must be attached to the bony structures in such a way as not to restrict motion in either joint, whether they move independently or simultaneously. The axes of motion of the ankle and subtalar joints lie in quite different planes, but the unique anatomic orientation of the ligament allows movement to occur in both joints.

Its fibular attachment to the tip of the lateral malleolus lies close to the axis of the ankle joint. Dorsiflexion and plantar flexion are therefore readily carried out without restriction by the ligament (Fig. 13.1).

From the tip of the malleolus the calcaneofibular ligament extends obliquely downward and medially to the lateral side of the calcaneus. The reason for this oblique course is to allow unrestricted movement in the subtalar joint. When projected onto the sagittal plane, the calcaneofibular ligament parallels the axis of the subtalar joint (see Appendix H for further details, and refer to Fig. 13.1). When projected onto a transverse plane the calcaneofibular ligament diverges from its attachment to the calcaneus to reach the tip of the malleolus (Fig. 13.2). Motion between the talus and calcaneus is around a single axis and unrestricted by the ligament since it lies on the surface of an imaginary cone. The central axis of the cone is

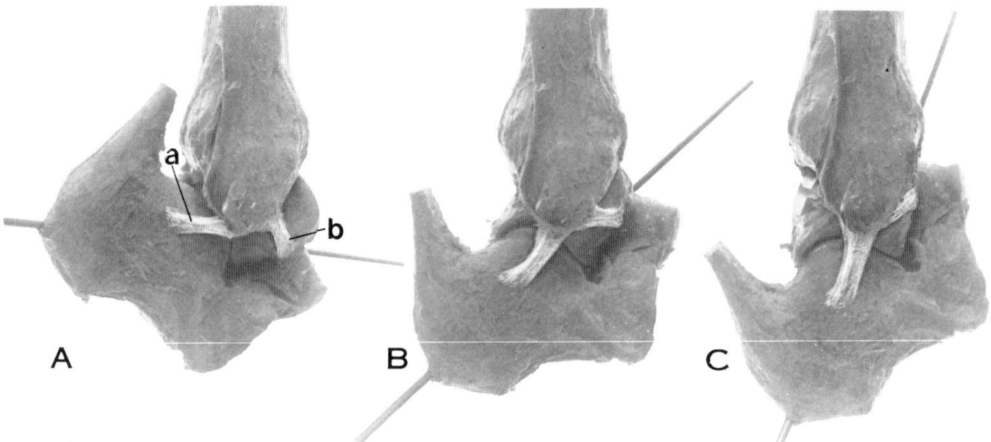

FIG. 13.1. Dissection of cadaver ankle showing lateral collateral ligaments. The ligaments have been bleached with H_2O_2 to increase their contrast. The calcaneofibular ligament (*a*) and the anterior talofibular ligament (*b*) are clearly shown. The posterior talofibular ligament is obscured by the overlying fibula. Note the change in positions of the ligaments in relation to the mortise of the ankle joint from full plantar flexion to full dorsiflexion. The angle between the anterior talofibular and calcaneofibular ligaments in this specimen is approximately 125°.

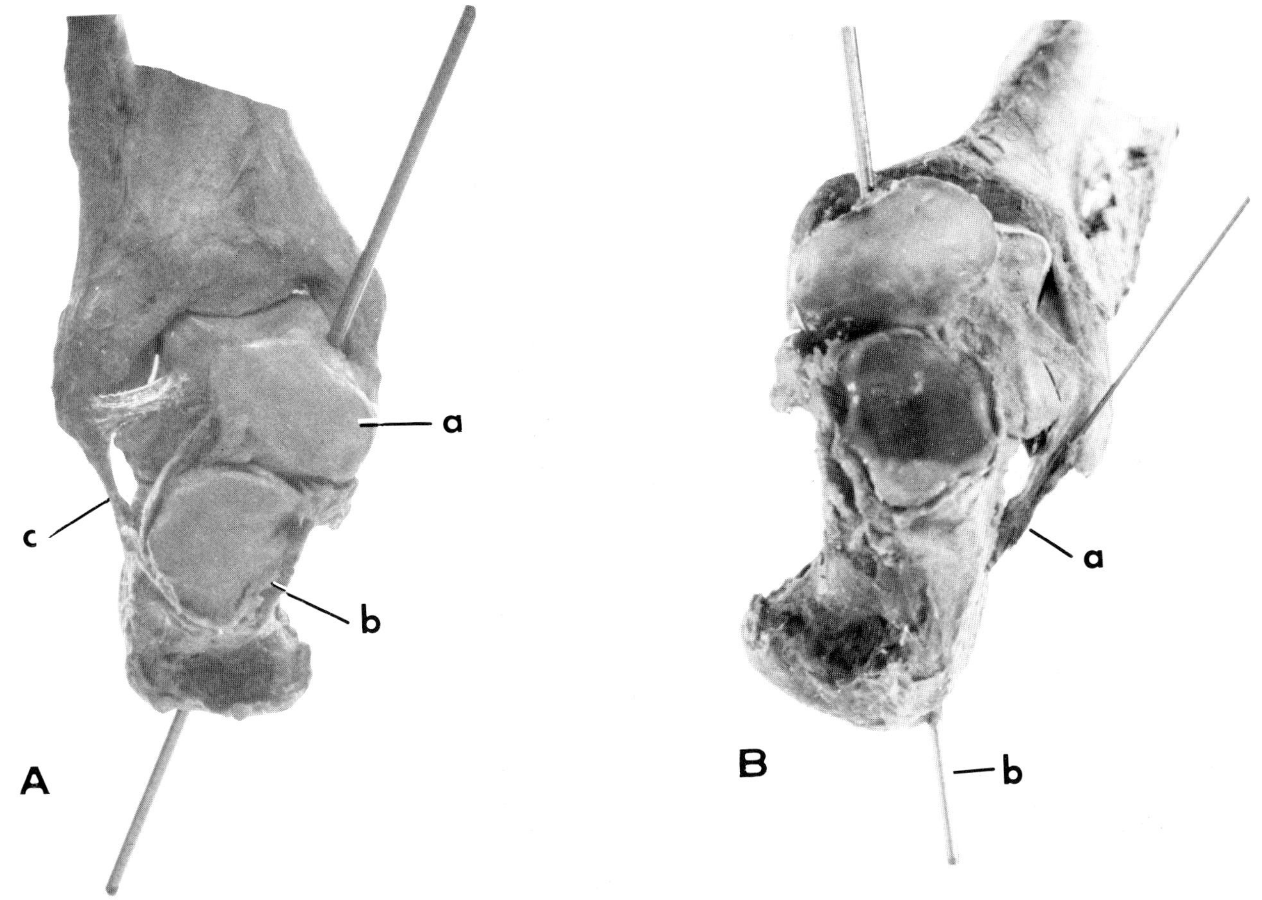

FIG. 13.2. Cadaver specimen. *A*, Anterior view. In the dissection the entire midfoot and forefoot have been removed. The talus (*a*) is seen articulating in the mortise above and with the calcaneus (*b*) below. The axis of the subtalar joint is represented by the 3-mm rod. The calcaneofibular ligament (*c*) is seen extending from the tip of the lateral malleolus downward and medially to the calcaneus. *B*, Same specimen viewed from below. A Kirschner wire (*a*) has been threaded through the fibers of the calcaneofibular ligament. Note the direction of the ligament extending from the malleolus to the lateral side of the calcaneus. If extended, the Kirschner wire would intersect at an acute angle the axis rod (*b*) within the lateral wall of the calcaneus.

the axis of movement of the subtalar joint. The arrangement is shown in Figure 13.3.

The inclination of the subtalar axis, particularly in the sagittal plane, has been shown to vary (see Fig. 9.1). This variation in the position of the subtalar axis appears unrelated to the variations in the ankle axis—scatter diagrams of individual measurements, at least, show no correlation. One would anticipate, therefore, that the anatomic relationships between the calcaneofibular ligament and the anterior and posterior talofibular ligaments would also show individual variations. The relationship between the calcaneofibular ligament and the anterior talofibular ligament appears to be of particular importance in maintaining stability of the talus in its mortise, and it warrants further discussion.

The angle between the calcaneofibular ligament and the anterior talofibular ligament was measured in two planes on 50 cadaver ankles (Appendix H). The average angles and the distribution of individual values are shown in Figure 13.4. Note that in the sagittal plane the angle between the two ligaments may vary from around 70 to 140°.

Attention is again directed to Figure 13.1. Several points require emphasis. Note that the calcaneofibular ligament retains its parallelism to the axis of the subtalar joint and that both the ligament and the axis alter their relationship to the ankle as this joint is moved. In plantar flexion both become horizontal and in dorsiflextion they approach a more vertical position. It is apparent that in dorsiflexion (Fig. 13.1*C*) the calcaneofibular ligament approaches a position in which it can serve as a true collateral ligament of the ankle joint and prevent tilting of the talus in its mortise. The anterior talofibular ligament can offer little resistance to talar tilt in this position since its

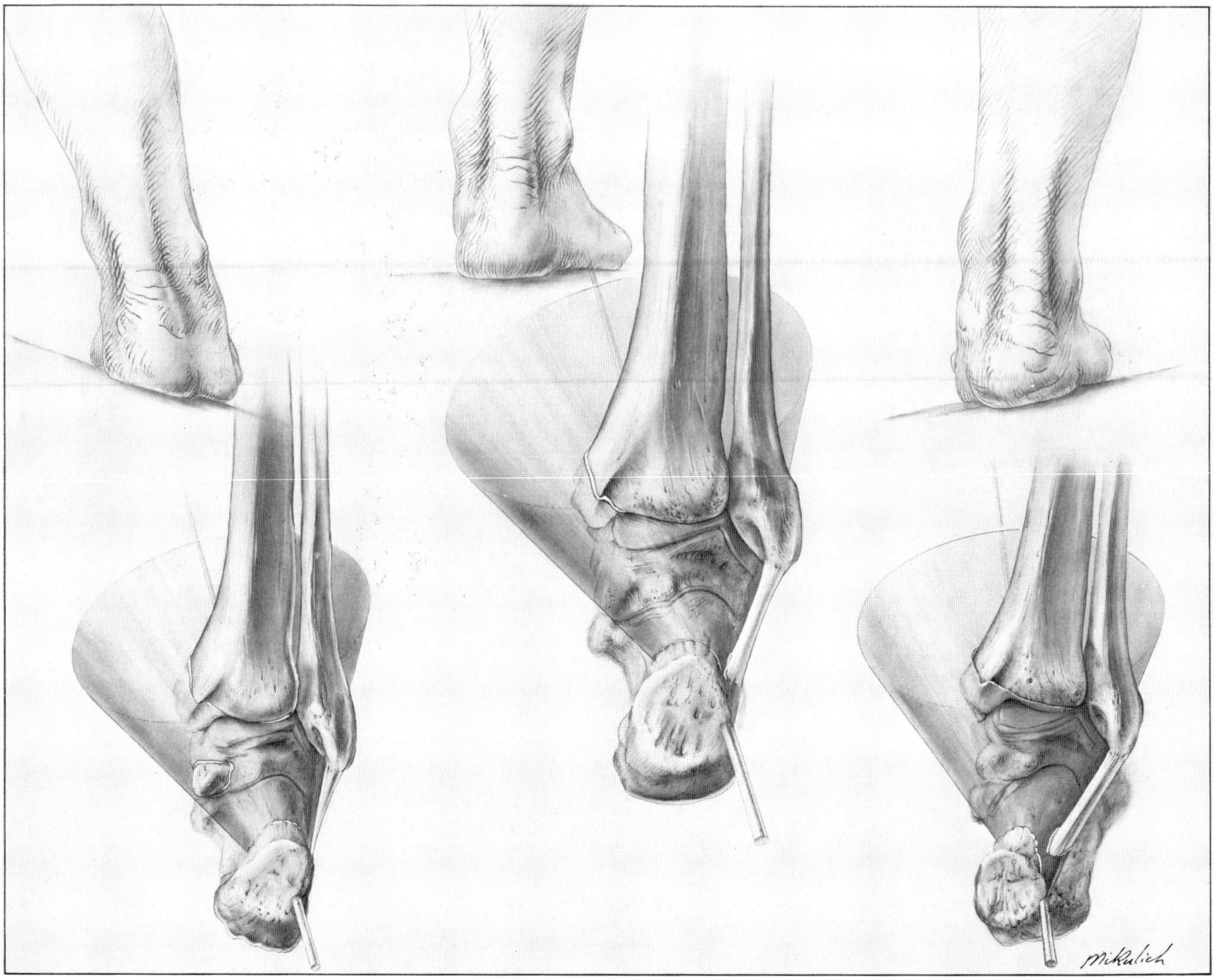

FIG. 13.3. Functional arrangement of calcaneofibular ligament. This drawing presents a concept which explains the mechanism in which free motion is permitted in the subtalar joint without restriction by the calcaneofibular ligament. An imaginary cone has been drawn around the axis of the subtalar joint. The calcaneofibular ligament is shown converging from its fibular attachment to the calcaneus. Since the ligament lies on the surface of the cone whose apex is the point of intersection of the functional extensions of the ligament and the axis of the subtalar joint, motion of the calcaneus under the talus is allowed without undue restriction from the ligament, which is merely displaced over the surface of the cone.

direction is upward and medialward. The reverse holds true in plantar flexion of the ankle (Fig. 13.1*A*). The calcaneofibular ligament has assumed a horizontal position and can offer little resistance to tilting of the talus. This role is dependent predominantly on the anterior talofibular ligament, which is now in a more vertical position.

It should be apparent that if the angle between the calcaneofibular and anterior talofibular ligaments, as projected onto the sagittal plane, is around 90°, the following situation will obtain. As the ankle is dorsiflexed and plantar flexed, one of the ligaments becomes progressively less able to prevent tilting by becoming more horizontal, while the other progressively assumes a more efficient vertical position. Therefore a definite reciprocal arrangement is present between the two ligaments which restricts talar tilt. However, should the angle between the two ligaments be more obtuse and approach an extreme value of 140°, plantar flexion of the ankle causes a problem. The calcaneofibular ligament, by becoming more horizontal, can provide little resistance to talar tilt at a time when the anterior talofibular ligament has not yet been displaced to a sufficiently vertical position to provide the necessary stability. Therefore there must exist a percentage of the population which should

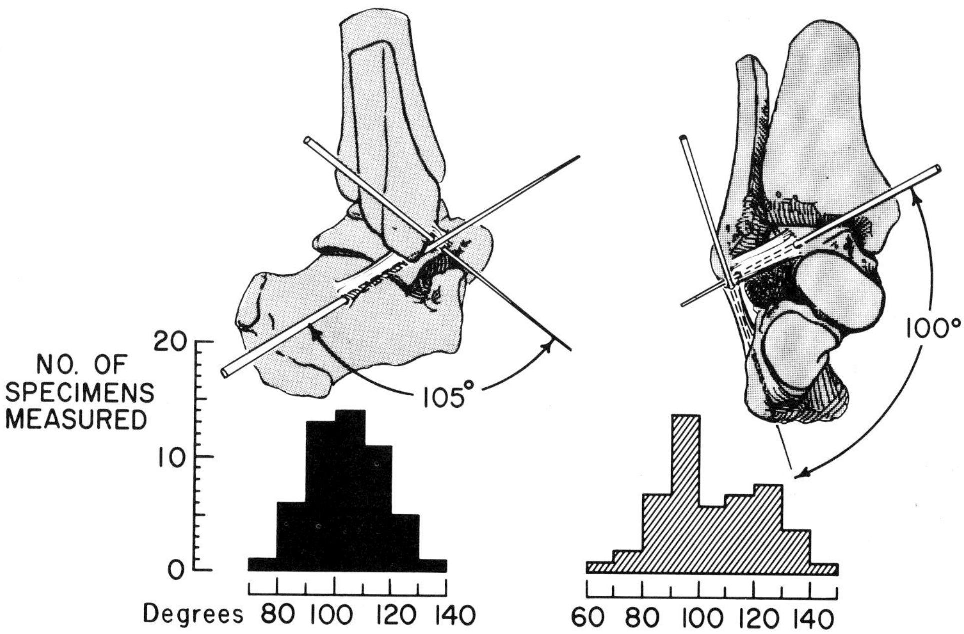

FIG. 13.4. Average angle between calcaneofibular and talofibular ligaments as measured in sagittal and coronal planes. Note the *histograms*, which indicate a considerable spread (70° in the sagittal and 90° in the coronal plane).

demonstrate instability of the talus in the mortise with plantar flexion.

Talar Tilt

A variable amount of talar tilt has been shown to occur normally within the population (Rubin and Witten, 1960). Using anthropometric data and assuming a normal distribution of angular values, we postulated that there would be approximately 10 to 15% of the population whose angle between the anterior talofibular and calcaneofibular ligaments would be greater than 120°. If the ankles of a random sample of individuals were subjected to standardized inversion stresses of the ankle in various positions of dorsiflexion, neutral position, and plantar flexion, it was anticipated that a greater number of individuals would show increased talar tilt with plantar flexion and that those that showed some talar tilt in the neutral position or in dorsiflexion would show an increase in talar tilt on plantar flexion. This procedure was carried out on 100 ankles (Appendix G). The results are shown graphically in Figure 13.5. It will be noted that both the number of subjects showing talar tilt and the degree of tilt increased with plantar flexion of the ankle.

An appreciation of the variations in the angle between the anterior talofibular and calcaneofibular ligaments and awareness of their changing positions in relation to the mortise of the ankle with dorsiflexion and plantar flexion of the ankle does more than merely explain talar tilt. It suggests the reason behind several additional clinical observations.

Stability of the Ankle

The impression that the ankle joint is more unstable in plantar flexion than in dorsiflexion probably corresponds to fact in a number of people. Increase in talar tilt with inversion stresses has been demonstrated. It now appears more reasonable to explain this instability on the basis of the individual arrangement of the collateral ligaments than on the belief that the instability is due to the narrower posterior portion of the trochlea occupying the wider anterior aspect of the mortise.

Sprains

An understanding of the changing roles of the components of the lateral collateral ligament in ankle stability, allows one to formulate what appears to be a rational basis to explain various types of sprains and propose methods of more accurately evaluating possible injuries to specific ligaments. The determination of whether or not the hypothesized procedures suggested here are valid will necessitate further clinical investigation. However, it appears reasonable to propose that forceful inversion of the ankle while it is plantar flexed will place the anterior talofibular ligament in a position in which it alone must withstand the imposed force. The calcaneofibular ligament, having been displaced into a more horizontal

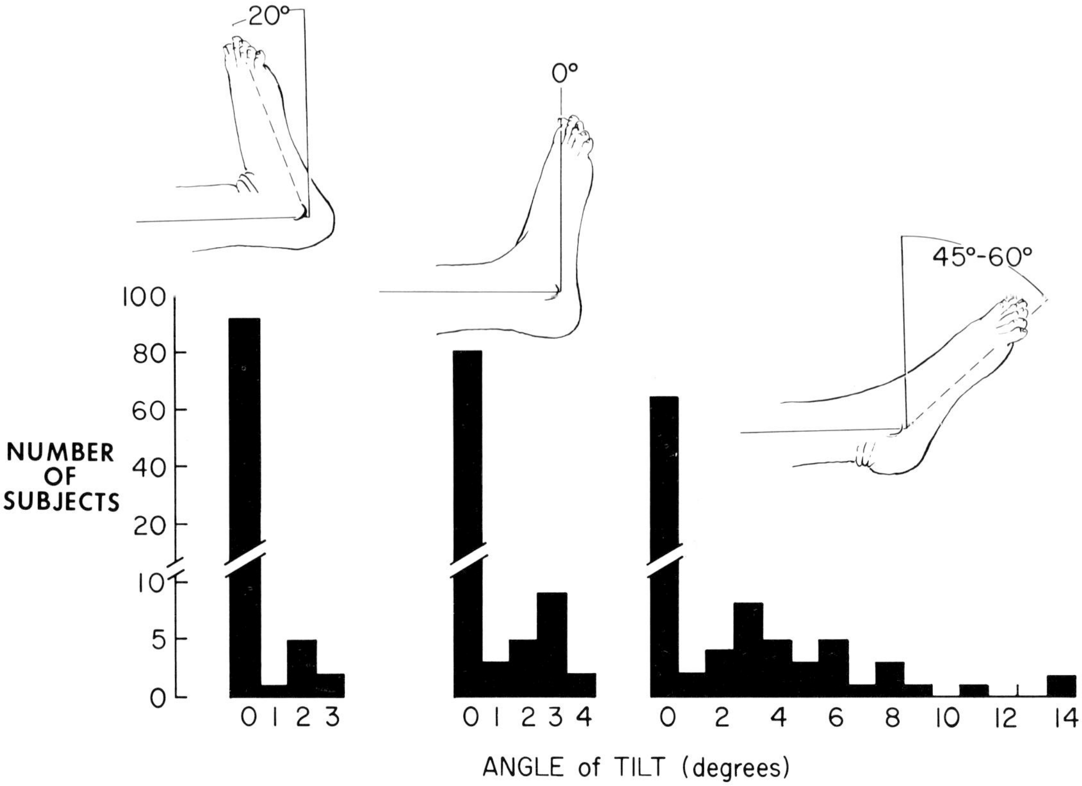

FIG. 13.5. *Histograms* showing talar tilt in 100 ankles. Note that with plantar flexion of the ankle both the number of ankles showing talar tilt and the degree of tilt were increased.

position, is less vulnerable. The reverse holds true if the ankle is in full dorsiflexion.

When checking for injuries to the collateral ligaments by stressing ankles, two factors should be kept in mind. If comparisons are being made between the injured and the sound ankle, care should be exercised to keep both ankles in the same amount of flexion or extension. Furthermore one may be able to distinguish whether the anterior talofibular ligament or the calcaneofibular ligament is torn by remembering the changing functional relationship of the two ligaments with changes in ankle position. In dorsiflexion the calcaneofibular ligament appears to function as the principal collateral ligament while the reverse occurs in plantar flexion.

Kelly (1952) expressed the opinion that common ankle sprains are the result of an exaggeration of one basic motion of the foot—either inversion or eversion. Inversion injuries are by far the more common. One has the impression that when an inversion injury is sustained the foot is more likely to be plantar flexed than in a neutral position or in dorsiflexion. The patient is usually recovering from a jump, turning while running, going down a steep grade, descending stairs, or twisting the ankle while wearing high heels. Rarely is the foot forcibly inverted when in dorsiflexion.

It has been demonstrated that in plantar flexion the anterior talofibular ligament plays the major role in restricting the tilting of the talus within the mortise. It is not surprising that this ligament should be the first to suffer injuries in minor sprains and is usually torn before injury to the calcaneofibular ligament. Staples (1975) reported that in 27 athletes who were explored surgically all had sustained tears of the anterior talofibular ligament while 19 had additional injuries to the calcaneofibular ligament.

Approximately one-half dozen surgical procedures have been proposed for the reconstruction of torn lateral collateral ligaments or for the stabilization of so-called weak ankles. All but one (Elmslie, 1934) of these procedures are based upon tenodesis of the peroneus brevis tendon and demonstrate a complete lack of understanding of the functional behavior of the components of the lateral collateral ligaments. In the tenodesis, the tendon extends from the fibula to the fifth metatarsal and its direction is in a plane at a right angle to the axis of motion of the subtalar joint. While it may provide stability to the ankle joint it must suppress subtalar motion.

Grice Extra-Articular Arthrodesis

In the Grice extra-articular arthrodesis, the surgeon should recall that the direction of the axis of the subtalar joint is downward and backward, making an angle with the sole of the foot of approximately 42° (p. 38). To provide maximal stabilization of the bone block, it should lie in a plane which is at a right angle to this axis. Therefore the bone block must be inclined upward and backward; otherwise any movement of the joint will tend to pry the graft from its bed.

Surgical Repair of Diastasis of the Tibiofibular Syndesmosis

This has been fully discussed in the text (pp. 6–7).

OSTEOCHONDRITIS DISSECANS AND OSTEOCHONDRAL FRACTURES

The increased ease with which the talus can be medially tilted in its mortise when the ankle is plantar flexed appears to explain the predilection of osteochondritis dissecans for the medial side of the trochlea. If it is assumed that the injury is due to a combined shear and compression of the articular surface of the trochlea, then with any degree of talar tilt these forces would be concentrated on the medial side. While the number of reported cases of osteochondritis dissecans in the world literature is small, the following distribution of the lesion in the ankle is of interest. Myhre (1939) reported three cases, all occurring on the medial side of the trochlea. Mensor and Melody (1941) reported a single case occurring on the medial side. Ray and Coughlin (1947) reported 13 cases, 10 of which occurred on the medial edge of the trochlea. Berndt and Harty (1959), in an extensive study of 214 transchondral fractures of the talus, reported lesions in 166 cases that involved the borders of the talus, 56.3% of which occurred on the medial side.

Smillie (1960) reported on lesions in 16 patients, 12 of which were on the medial side; he added that, of the four on the lateral side, two were "undoubtedly osteochondral fractures" and thus not true cases of osteochondritis dissecans. Junge and von Känel (1964) reported their findings on 184 football players. Of those demonstrating osteochondritic lesions, the medial border of the trochlea was involved four times more frequently than was the lateral border. Gustilo and Gordon (1968) reported on 10 patients, but the text does not clearly state whether the lesion was located on the medial or the lateral side. However, the three x-ray reproductions used to depict typical lesions show these to be located on the medial side of the talus.

On theoretical grounds based upon the material presented here, one would expect that lesions on the medial edge of the talus would result from compression forces due to talar tilt and that these may occur without necessarily requiring rupture of the lateral collateral ligaments. Lesions on the lateral side would require rupture of the lateral ligaments and avulsion of the lateral edge of the trochlea by contact with the inner facet of the fibular malleolus (Berndt and Harty, 1959).

INTERNAL PROSTHESES

The surgical replacement of human joints with plastic or metallic prostheses is becoming more widespread. Following the successful utilization of internal prostheses in diseased hip joints, attempted replacement of other joints has naturally followed. At the present time experience has shown that internal prostheses for the knee and shoulder are far from satisfactory. This appears to be the result of mechanical designs which have been based upon inadequate biomechanical data.

Recently, prosthetic replacement of the ankle has been attempted. Buchholz (1974) employed a cylindrical replacement, with the axis of the cylinder being horizontal, and Smith (1973, 1974) utilized a ball-and-socket type of prosthesis. A review of the intimate functional relationships between the talocrural and subtalar joints would seem to indicate that both types may be applicable in specific situations. Theoretically, the retention of normal motion in the subtalar joint would suggest that a prosthesis of cylindrical or conical shape would prove adequate. However, if both ankle and subtalar motion is lost, then a ball-and-socket type of prosthesis would seem to be required.

In any case, orthopaedic surgeons who are considering the design of a new ankle prosthesis or contemplating the insertion of such a device should carefully reflect upon the functional interrelationship between the ankle and the subtalar joints.

TORSION IN THE CALCANEAL TENDON

All textbooks agree that the principal action of the triceps surae is to cause plantar flexion of the foot. If the only function of the calcaneal tendon is to transmit muscular forces from the triceps surae to the calcaneus and if the motion produced is purely one of flexion and extension of the foot in a vertical plane, the following question immediately arises. Why do the fibers of the tendon undergo a spiral twist in their course from their muscular origin to their insertion into the calcaneus?

Most textbooks of anatomy fail to mention this spiral arrangement. Whereas in two texts the artist has clearly shown the twist in the tendon in accompanying illustrations (Henle, 1871; Rauber-Kopsch, 1968), no description of this phenomenon appears in the texts. Among the more modern texts, only Morris (1966) states, "The bundles of fibers of the tendon take a slightly spiral course." Comparative anatomists (Parsons, 1894; Jones, 1944) have reported that the spiral arrangement of the fibers is not exclusively a human characteristic but is even more apparent in other mammals. Furthermore, the spiral arrangement has been demonstrated to be present in the newborn human (Reck, 1971; Clark, 1972).

The twist in the calcaneal tendon has presented a difficulty for the surgeon attempting to tenotomize it. Acting upon the belief that the fibers are parallel and straight, he makes hemisections at different levels on opposite sides of the tendon, but these fail to cut all fibers and the proximal and distal segments do not slip past one another readily. This surgical difficulty has led to repeated investigations by surgeons of the precise internal arrangement of the fibers comprising the tendon (Alezais, 1899; White, 1943; Cummins *et al.*, 1946; Bíró and Tarsoly, 1967). There appears to be complete agreement among surgeons and anatomists who have carefully investigated the subject, that there exists in man, as in other mammals, a spiral twist to the fibers which constitute the calcaneal tendon. While the amount of twist varies, the direction is the same in all. The twist is such that the fibers comprising the posterior surface of the tendon run from its medial side toward the lateral side of the calcaneus. The fibers comprising the anterior surface run in a reverse direction.

Before proceeding further with any discussion concerning the twist of the calcaneal tendon, certain anatomic facts must be emphasized. Tensile forces transmitted from the leg to the foot through the calcaneal tendon must pass through two joints, the ankle and the subtalar joints. In this process moments are developed around the axes of both joints. However, it should be recalled that the axes of the two joints are quite differently oriented; the ankle axis basically permits dorsiflexion and plantar flexion of the foot, while the subtalar joint permits inversion and eversion of the foot. For the sake of clarity, it appears expedient to discuss the action of the calcaneal tendon upon the ankle and subtalar joints as if they were independent events.

The magnitude of the moments depends upon the lengths of their respective lever arms. The lever arm for plantar flexion of the ankle joint is readily recognized as the perpendicular distance between the axis of the ankle and the insertion of the calcaneal tendon on the calcaneus. This varies about an average of approximately 5 cm. That an inversion moment at the subtalar joint may be developed through tension in the calcaneal tendon is not so apparent and requires further consideration. The effective lever arm is the perpendicular distance between the axis of the subtalar joint and the insertion of the calcaneal tendon. However, two difficulties immediately arise in attempting to secure such a measurement. The first is that the tendon becomes flattened in its anteroposterior dimension as it approaches its insertion. The average width of the tendon as measured in 102 cadaver specimens was found to be 20 mm. In addition, this dimension lies in a plane almost perpendicular to the direction of the subtalar axis. The question immediately arises at what point in the tendon one should assume the forces to be concentrated since this point should be used for the measurement of the effective lever arm. The second difficulty arises when one considers the variations in the point of emergence of the subtalar axis on the lateral side of the calcaneus and its relationship to the calcaneal tendon. This was studied in 102 cadaver specimens (Appendix K). It will be seen that in half of the specimens the axis of the subtalar joint passed within 2 mm of the lateral edge of the calcaneal tendon (Fig. 13.6). In the remaining specimens the axis passed a greater distance either lateral or medial to the lateral edge of the tendon. Thus regardless of what one assumes to be the point of application of the force of the calcaneal tendon, the effective lever arm for inversion of the heel must vary considerably from individual to individual. However, in the majority of feet, tension transmitted through the calcaneal tendon will produce an inversion moment, although the magnitude of the moment may be almost negligible in some persons and considerable in others. In a small number of persons (less than 10%) tension in the tendon may produce eversion of the heel.

Inversion of the heel normally occurs simultaneously with plantar flexion and may be seen in any normal person (Fig. 13.7). This means that movement is occurring in both ankle and subtalar joints. It appears reasonable to assume that an anatomic arrangement obtains in the fibers of the calcaneal

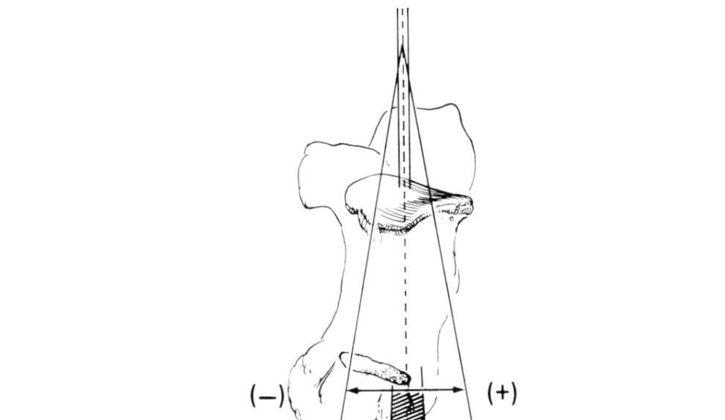

FIG. 13.6. Relation of subtalar axis to insertion of calcaneal tendon. Note that in approximately one-half of 102 specimens the axis passed within 2 mm of the lateral edge of the tendon.

tendon that permits these combined movements to occur without undue tensions being placed upon individual fibers of the tendon or without requiring any internal slippage between the fibers within the tendon.

An explanation for the presence of a spiral arrangement of the fibers of the calcaneal tendon seems to emerge when one considers carefully the movements that occur about the oblique axes of the ankle and subtalar joints. Since several factors are simultaneously involved, a written description becomes exceedingly complicated. Therefore, wooden models are used. The most simple mechanical arrangements are demonstrated first. Additional factors are added sequentially until the final model approximates the actual anatomic situation that exists in the human ankle and foot. The reader is asked to study the photographs of the models carefully. The legends call attention to the pertinent facts that are illustrated by the models.

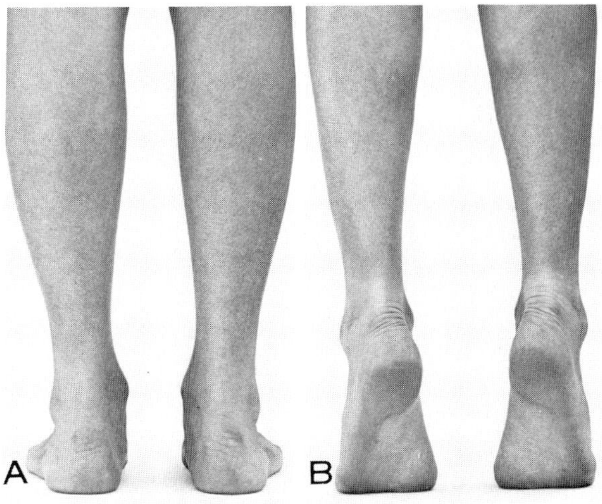

FIG. 13.7. Combined plantar flexion and inversion of heels. *A*, Subject standing. *B*, Subject on tiptoe. Note that plantar flexion is accompanied by inversion of the heels. On plantar flexion the presence of skin creases, which appear on the medial sides of the leg just above the heel, indicates that the distance between the medial side of the heel and the leg has been lessened as compared with the lateral side.

The first model has been constructed with a simple hinge representing the ankle joint connecting the leg and the foot (Fig. 13.8). The orientation of the hinge is horizontal and perpendicular to the sagittal plane and midline of the foot. Two wires have been added to represent the medial and lateral edges of the calcaneal tendon. Arrows have been fixed to each wire to reveal any unequal excursions between the medial and lateral wires. Note that in this situation there is equal excursion of the wires from full dorsiflexion to full plantar flexion.

The situation depicted in the first model, however, rarely occurs. The axis of the ankle joint is directed laterally and downward. In the second model (Fig. 13.9) the ankle axis is inclined laterally and downward at 20°, but it remains perpendicular to the midline of the foot. Dorsiflexion and plantar flexion are again depicted. Note that such an orientation of the ankle axis results in only a minimal difference in the excursion of the wires. In the third model (Fig. 13.10), the axis has been rotated to provide 21° of external tibial torsion. The axis is now directed laterally, downward, and posteriorly to more nearly approximate the average position of the ankle axis. Now dorsiflexion and plantar flexion necessitate a slightly greater excursion of the medial wire. If the fibers of the calcaneal tendon were straight and

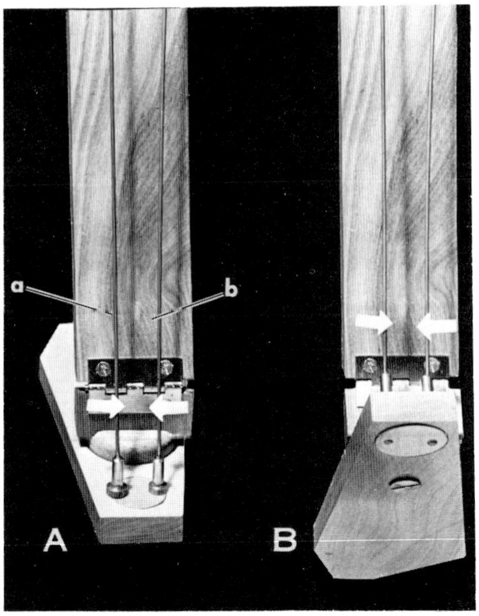

FIG. 13.8. Basic model to be utilized in demonstrating effects of twist in calcaneal tendon. The model is similar to the models previously employed and consists of a vertical member that represents the leg and a horizontal member roughly shaped to resemble a foot. The model depicts a right leg and foot and is viewed from the back. Two parallel wires have been attached to the heel portion of the wooden foot by means of ball-and-socket joints. The wires are intended to represent the lateral edge (*a*) and the medial edge (*b*) of the calcaneal tendon. An *arrow* has been fixed to each wire to show any unequal excursion of the wires. In this model the hinge representing the ankle joint has been oriented to lie horizontal and perpendicular to the sagittal plane of the leg and to the midline of the foot. Note that motion of the foot from dorsiflexion (*A*) to plantar flexion (*B*) results in equal excursions of the two wires.

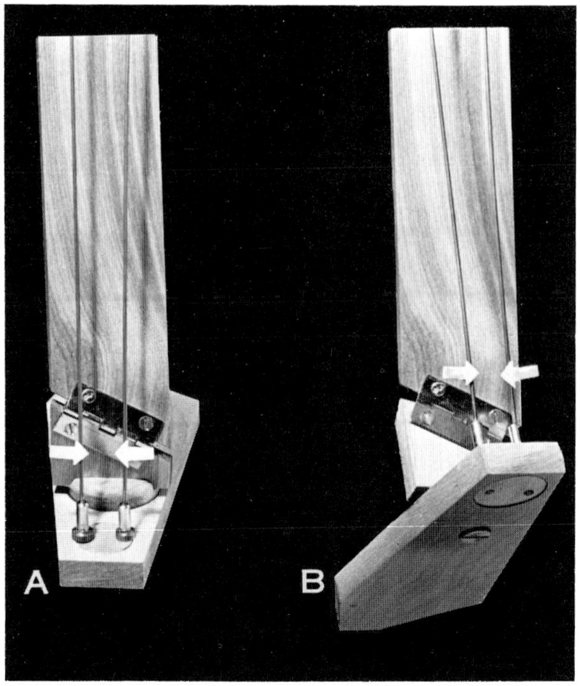

FIG. 13.9. Effect of oblique ankle joint axis. In this model the hinge has been oriented so as to incline laterally and downward while remaining perpendicular to the midline of the foot. The angle of inclination of the hinge is 20°. This angulation has been chosen because it approximates the maximal value for the inclination of the ankle axis as revealed in the anthropometric studies and because it will result in the exaggeration of any unequal excursions that may occur in the two wires. Note that from dorsiflexion (*A*) to plantar flexion (*B*) there has been only a slight difference in the excursion of the wires.

parallel as represented by the wires in the model, some longitudinal slippage between the medial and lateral fibers of the tendon would be required.

In the fourth model (Fig. 13.11) the hinge representing the ankle joint has been omitted, but a hinge representing the subtalar axis has been substituted. The axis of the hinge forms an angle of 45° with the leg and plane of the foot and in the horizontal plane the axis has been inclined posterolaterally by 23° to the midline of the foot. This approximates the average orientation of the subtalar axis (p. 38). Movement from full eversion to full inversion of the foot now causes a marked difference in the excursion of the two wires.

In the fifth model (Fig. 13.12), both ankle and subtalar joints have been included and are represented by two crossed hinges, welded together in an approximately average relationship. The fibers of the calcaneal tendon, as depicted by the wires, run straight and parallel. If this is the situation, motion from dorsiflexion-eversion to plantar flexion-inversion, which has been shown to occur simultaneously (see Fig. 13.7), would require the medial side of the tendon to move faster and through a greater excursion than the lateral fibers. This would necessitate a marked longitudinal slippage between individual fibers comprising the tendon, an unlikely and unnatural situation.

If longitudinal slippage between the medially and laterally placed fibers of the calcaneal tendon does occur, then a needle passed horizontally through the tendon should show a tilt as the foot is plantar flexed. However, this does not happen. Figure 13.13 is a photograph of a subject in whom a hypodermic needle has been inserted through the calcaneal tendon. As the subject rises on her toes the needle moves upward but remains horizontal. This appears to prove that equal excursion of all fibers of the calcaneal tendon

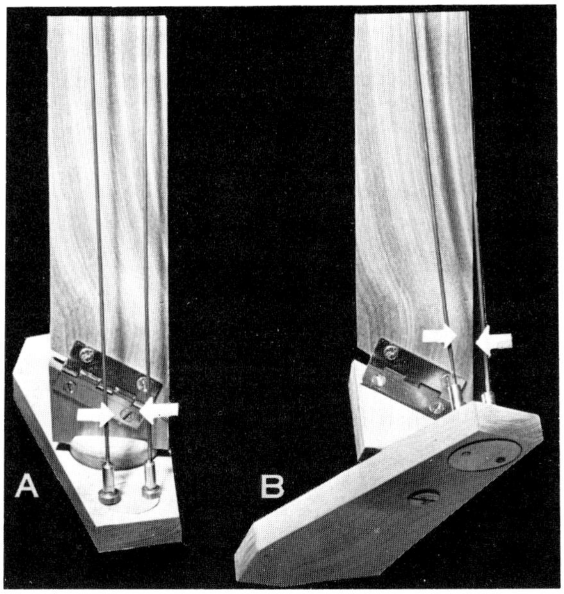

FIG. 13.10. Added effect of tibial torsion. The orientation of the hinge has been altered from the previous model by adding 20° of external tibial torsion. The hinge is now not only inclined laterally and downward as in the previous model but has been rotated laterally and posteriorly. The effect of such an orientation of the hinge now causes an unequal excursion of the two wires. The medial wire undergoes a greater excursion than the lateral wire.

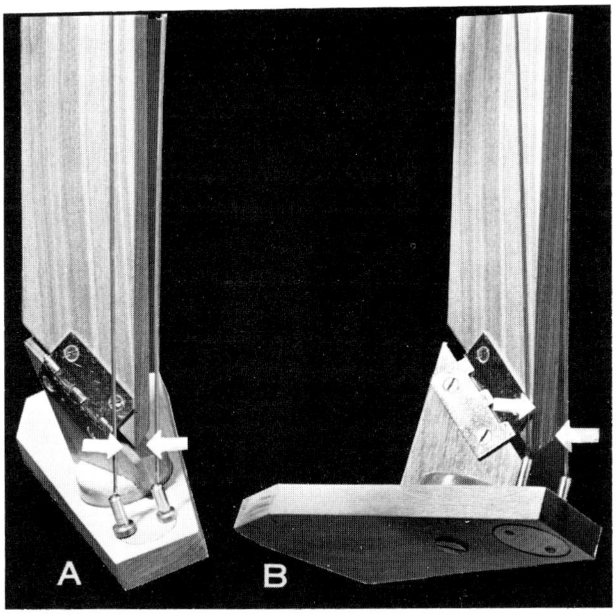

FIG. 13.11. Effect of subtalar axis. The ankle hinge has been replaced by a hinge representing the subtalar axis. The hinge is oriented to be at an angle of 45° to both the leg and the foot and inclined posterolaterally 23° from the midline of the foot. Movement of the foot is now one of eversion (*A*) and inversion (*B*). Note that such movement causes a marked difference in the excursion of the two wires; the medial wire is forced to move through a greater distance than is the lateral wire.

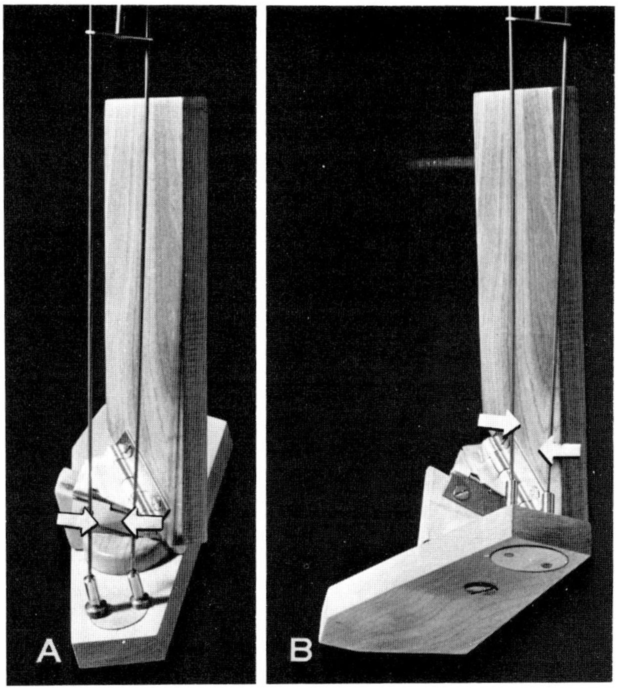

FIG. 13.12. Combined motions of dorsiflexion-eversion and plantar flexion-inversion. Two hinges are incorporated in the model, one representing the ankle joint and the other the subtalar joint. *A*, Dorsiflexion of ankle combined with eversion of foot. *B*, Plantar flexion combined with inversion of foot. The wires representing the medial and lateral fibers of the calcaneal tendon are parallel. Note that the medial wire undergoes a greater excursion than does the lateral wire.

has taken place and to rule out the improbable occurrence of internal slippage between fibers of the tendon.

In Figure 13.14, the wires representing the calcaneal tendon have been twisted approximately 100°. Such a twist directs the medial wire laterally as it approaches its attachment to the foot and the lateral wire in a reverse direction. This is precisely the direction of the twist that has been described by surgeons and comparative anatomists to be present in man and other mammals. Note that the presence of such a twist results in an almost equal excursion of the two wires from dorsiflexion with eversion to plantar flexion with inversion. It appears that the simple expedient of incorporating a twist in the calcaneal tendon equalizes the excursion of all the fibers comprising the tendon and eliminates the necessity for any longitudinal slippage between individual fibers during the combined movements of dorsiflexion with eversion and plantar flexion with inversion.

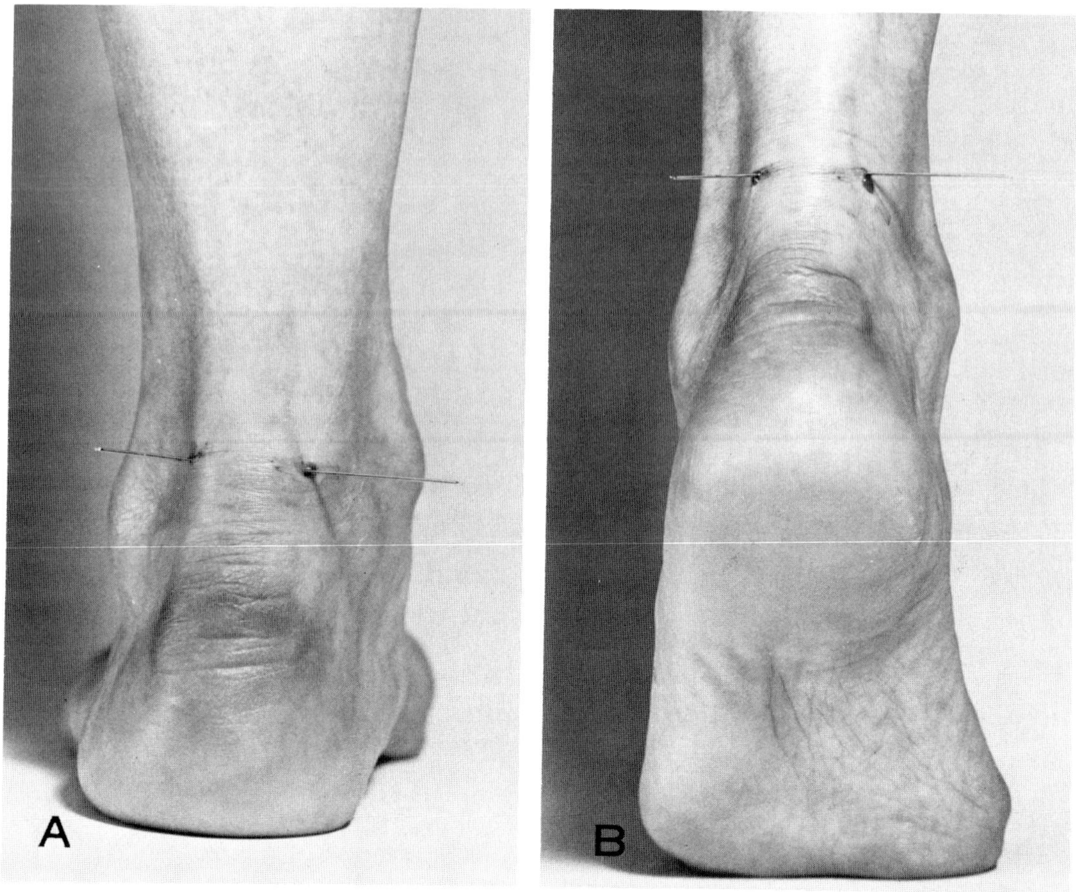

FIG. 13.13. Needle through calcaneal tendon. In *A* a #20 spinal puncture needle, with its base removed, has been inserted through the left calcaneal tendon. In *B* the subject rises on tiptoe. Note that the needle does not tilt but remains in a horizontal plane.

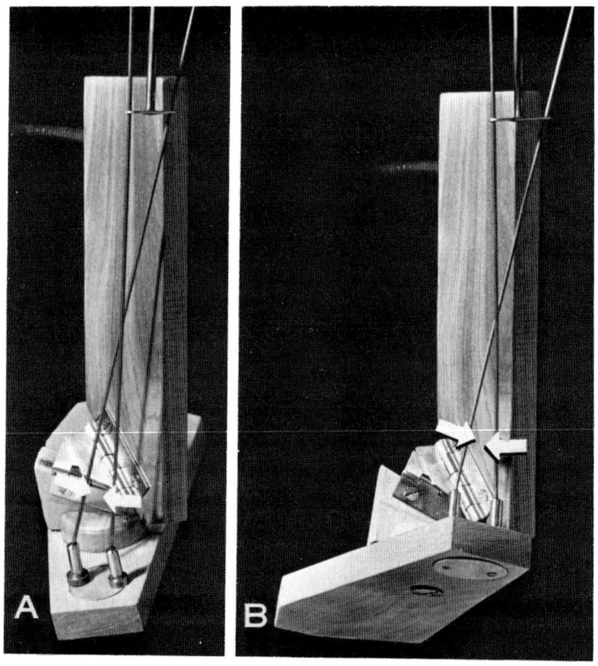

FIG. 13.14. Effect of twisting wires. The same model is employed and the same motions are shown as in Figure 13.12. However, the wires have been twisted approximately 10° at their attachment to the foot. The medial wire now runs laterally as it approaches the heel and the lateral wire runs medially. Note that such an arrangement equalizes the excursion of the two wires.

appendices A–K

INTRODUCTION

Any comparative study of human joints designed to determine the extent of individual variations in the location of axes of motion and to detect minor differences in movement is beset with numerous difficulties. This is especially true if the investigations are restricted to the study of living subjects. Direct inspection of the moving articular surfaces is impossible without surgical exposure. X-rays or cine-x-rays project the movement onto a single plane and thus make accurate measurements almost impossible. The use of externally applied mechanical measuring devices requires firm skeletal attachment of the devices; this is difficult to obtain without pin or screw fixation directly to the articulating bones. While this procedure has been used with success in limited studies, it is not applicable, for obvious reasons, to the collection of a series of observations large enough to be statistically significant.

For these reasons, the only adequate sources of material for the projected statistical study appear to be cadaver specimens (which are continuously available from the anatomic dissecting laboratories), supplemented with freshly amputated specimens.

The use of embalmed cadaver joints entails certain difficulties. The addition of formaldehyde to the embalming fluid results in some shrinkage of soft tissues, amounting, however, to less than 3% (Schultz, 1919), and this amount of shrinkage occurring in the articular cartilage is not likely to lead to gross errors. Furthermore, values obtained from measurement of unembalmed specimens and from repeat measurements of the same specimens after formalin fixation showed no measurable differences with use of the techniques employed in this study.

More serious than shrinkage is the problem of fixation of the soft tissues which results from the loss of elasticity incurred during embalming. Inelastic soft tissues either restrict motion or impose abnormal displacements on the moving joint surfaces. For the study of joint motion it is therefore necessary to remove all capsular and ligamentous structures to permit full and free movement of the joint. Then the only remaining factors which can influence joint motion are the configuration of the articular surfaces and the effects of friction. To simulate normal motion, the surfaces must be held in close contact by a constantly applied pressure. While one component of the joint is rigidly held in some type of clamp, the other component must be free to rotate and slide in all three planes of space, restricted solely by the configurations of the articulating surfaces. The pressure holding the surfaces together must be a force which is constant through the entire range of motion of the joint, and its direction must always remain perpendicular to the area of contact between the two apposing articular surfaces. The two surfaces are never completely congruent, and a force directed tangentially will result in abnormal displacements of the articular surfaces.

The constantly applied pressure must also be adjusted to simulate friction in the joint. The coefficient of friction of joints is increased in embalmed specimens. Although the surfaces glide with surprising smoothness, they appear to react in accordance with the law of dry friction: the greater the pressure between the surfaces, the greater the force required to move them. Experience indicates that a force of between 4.5 and 9 kg is optimal. A force of less than 4 kg permits abnormal movement, and repetitive motions may yield slightly different measurements. Forces in excess of 9 kg lead to momentary sticking of the articular surfaces, so that smooth repetitive movement is difficult to obtain.

The design and construction of adequate joint measurement devices (articulators) presents many problems. Since each joint must be considered separately, a specific articulator must be designed to hold it and to measure its motion. In addition, the bone holders should be adaptable to both right- and left-sided specimens as well as to a variety of sizes. The points and types of fixation of the specimens of the bones have to be selected so as not to interfere with the movements to be studied or injure the articular surfaces of adjacent joints, which are preserved for further studies.

The design of each articulator was revised many times before the instrument would perform satisfactorily and fulfill all the criteria set forth in the previous paragraphs.

In addition to the articulators, various accessory apparatus were developed. These consisted of special goniometers, locators for determining functional axes of motion, and guides for drill holes which received stainless steel rods to simulate the functional axes. Special devices to measure the contours and shapes of articular surfaces were constructed or purchased.

Since each procedure presented different problems and required individualized apparatus, it is necessary to discuss the measuring devices and procedural techniques separately. Although the instruments are relatively simple, a written description of each would be difficult; therefore, photographs with descriptive legends will be used. These will be presented sequentially, illustrating each procedural step and the manner in which each device operates.

appendix A

method of locating the ankle axis and obtaining various measurements

The ankle joint may be described as a typical hinge joint, although there is disagreement as to whether it has a single or a changing axis. Determination of its axis was accomplished as follows.

Step 1. The tibia is fixed firmly in the clamp of the articulator. The fibula remains free so that lateral or rotatory displacements of this bone can be detected during movement of the joint (Fig. A-1).

Step 2. The disarticulated talus is fixed in its holder (Fig. A-2).

Step 3. The talus in its holder is inverted and articulated within the ankle mortise (Fig. A-3).

Step 4. The articulator, supporting the talus in its mortise, is assembled. Accuracy of fit and smoothness of motion are checked while the joint is carried through its full range of motion (Fig. A-4).

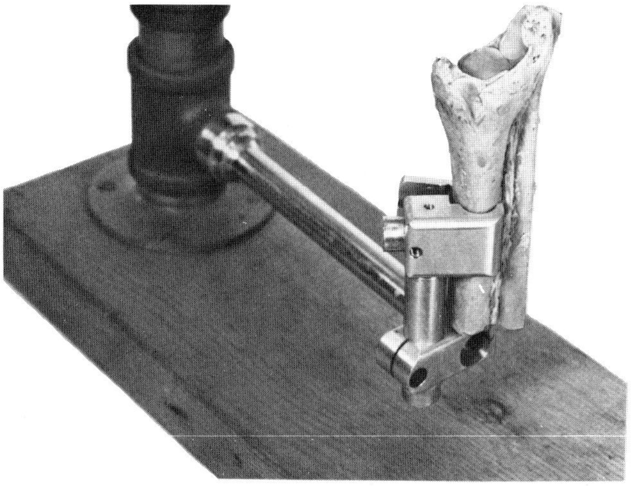

FIG. A-1. Tibia held rigidly in clamp on articulator, with fibula free so that any movement can be detected.

Step 5. The adjustable axis locator is manipulated

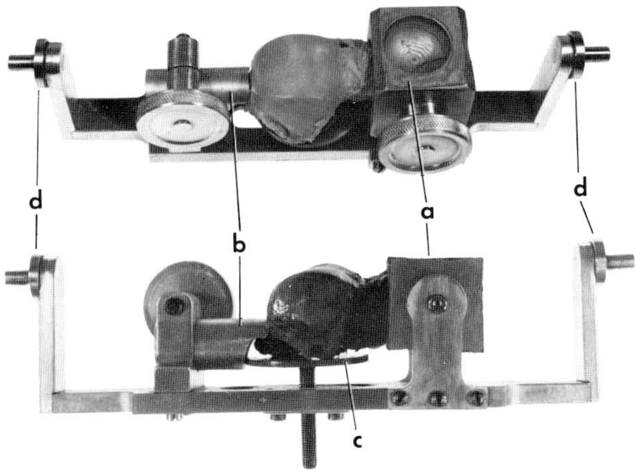

FIG. A-2. Holder for talus. *a*, Rotating block with hemispherical concavities of four different dimensions for reception of head of talus, which varies in size; *b*, adjustable tube provided with lip to fix nonarticular posterior ledge of talus; *c*, movable platform to provide three-point fixation of talus; *d*, arms supporting pins for attachment to articulator. The centers of the pins are on approximately the same level as the surface of the trochlea. This ensures stability of the holder when placed in the articulator and also permits the holder to swivel freely and maintain lateral contact between the articular surfaces.

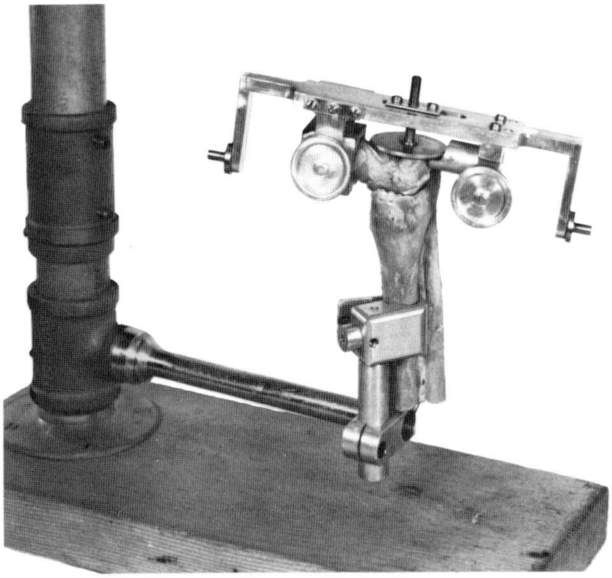

FIG. A-3. Inversion and articulation of talus in its holder within ankle mortise.

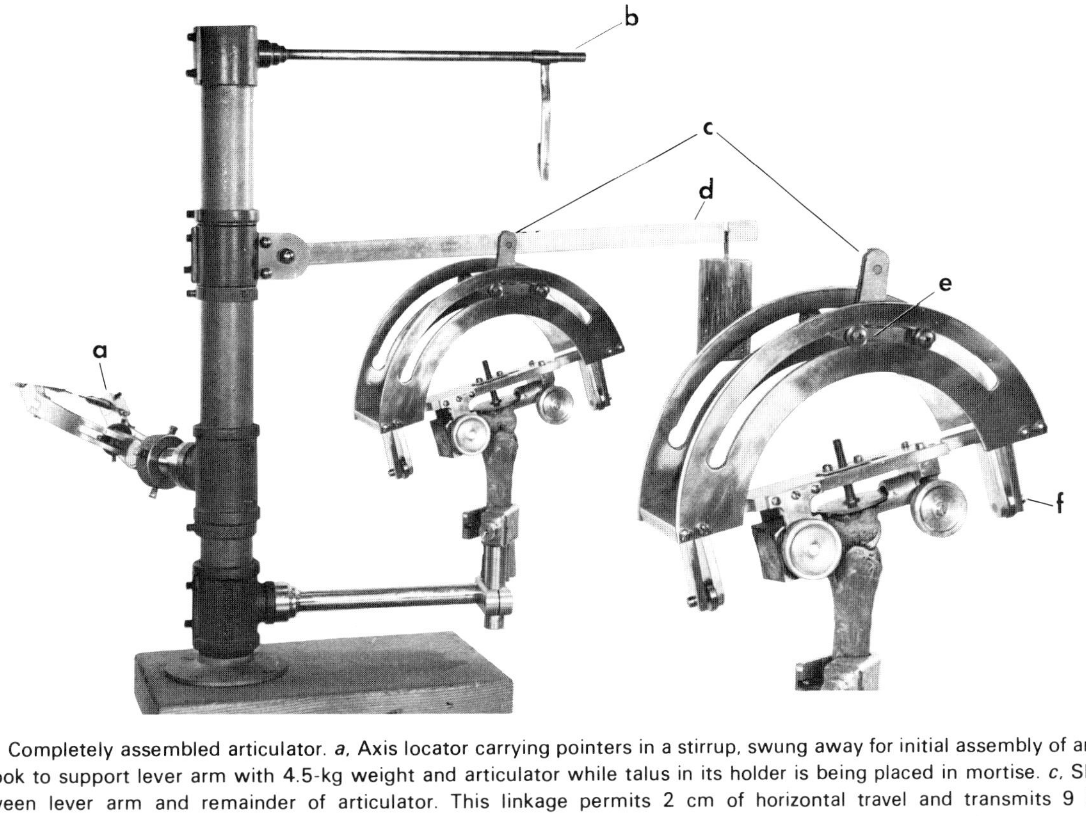

FIG. A-4. Completely assembled articulator. *a*, Axis locator carrying pointers in a stirrup, swung away for initial assembly of articulator. *b*, Arm with hook to support lever arm with 4.5-kg weight and articulator while talus in its holder is being placed in mortise. *c*, Short linkage placed between lever arm and remainder of articulator. This linkage permits 2 cm of horizontal travel and transmits 9 kg of force perpendicular to the articulating surfaces of the bones during movement of the talus in its mortise. *d*, Lever arm, acting as compression bar, supporting 4.5-kg weight. *e*, Carriage, traveling on double circular track, permitting rotation of talus in its mortise. A bearing placed between the short linkage and the carriage allows free rotation of the carriage in a horizontal plane. *f*, Slotted bars to receive pins on talus holder, allowing it to swivel within mortise.

until the pointers are directed toward the points on the medial and lateral sides of the talus which demonstrate minimal displacement as the talus is rotated in the articulator from full flexion to full extension. The pointer on one side is located, then pressed into the cortex of the bone to fix it firmly. The axis locator is manipulated on the opposite side of the bone until its pointer is over a point of minimal motion. It is also pushed into the cortex. This determines an external axis (two pointers) about which the talus must move. The accuracy of the location of the axis is now checked by rotating the talus and observing the degree of contact between the articulating surfaces of the joint (Fig. A-5).

Step 6. All adjustments on the axis locator are rigidly fixed.

Step 7. Motion of the talus in its mortise is again checked to confirm the accuracy of the positioning pointers.

Step 8. The pointers are removed from the stirrup of the axis locator and replaced with drill guides, and a 3-mm hole is drilled through the talus (Fig. A-6).

Step 9. The drill is removed and replaced with a stainless steel rod (15 cm in length and 3 mm in diameter). The talus is disengaged from its holder, and the upper portion of the articulator, with its 9 kg

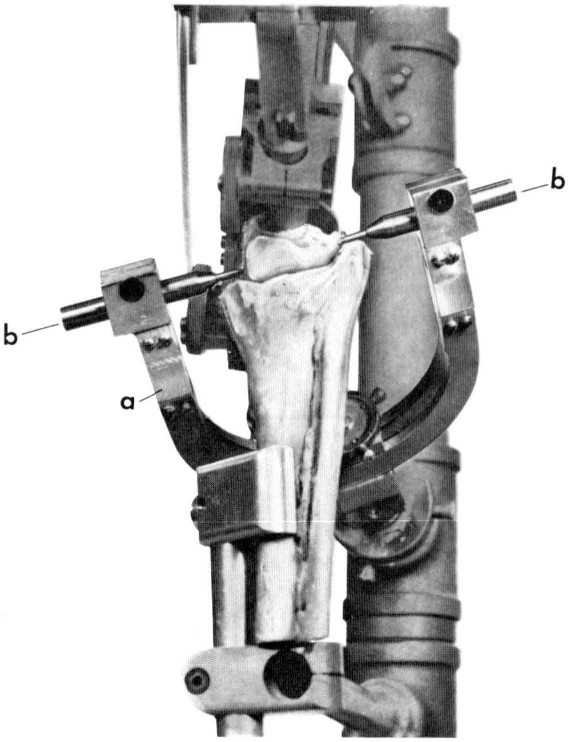

FIG. A-5. End view of carriage, with axis locator in place. *a*, Stirrup, adjustable in all directions and carrying sharpened pointers. *b*, Pointers carried on 10-mm stainless steel rods to assure rigidity.

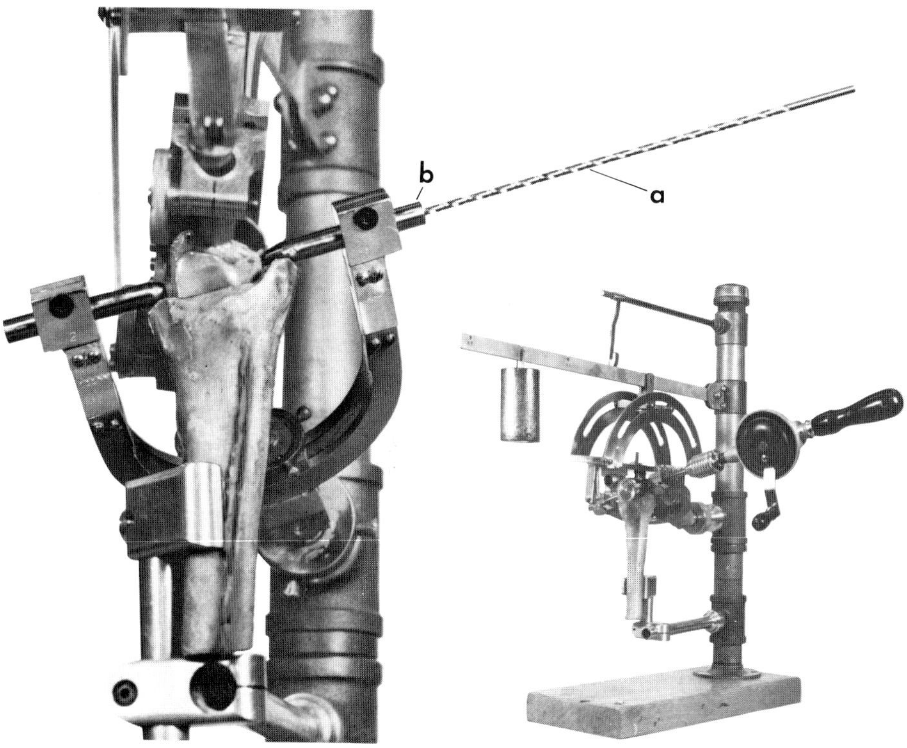

FIG. A-6. Establishment of rigid axis. *a*, 3-mm stainless steel drill; *b*, hollow drill guides. The *smaller figure* shows drilling of the hole through the talus controlled by the hollow drill guides that replaced the pointers in the axis locator stirrup.

of force, is removed. The movement of the talus in the mortise is checked for maximal contact of the articular surfaces and smoothness of movement; the talus is now forced to rotate around the fixed axis determined by the 3-mm stainless steel rod held rigidly in its stirrup (Fig. A-7).

Step 10. The measurement of the angle between the plafond of the mortise and the midline of the tibia required the use of a special goniometer. The plafond is concave in an anteroposterior plane and it has a slight medial elevation. To determine a plane which would closely correspond to the average inclination of the plafond, two hemidisks fixed to a movable slide were added to the goniometer. The isolated goniometer is shown in Figure A-8 and its application is shown in Figure A-9. Without loosening the axis locator with the drill guides, the stainless steel pin is withdrawn and the talus is removed from the mortise. The angle between the surface of the mortise (plafond) and the center line of the tibia is measured with the goniometer (Fig. A-10).

Step 11. The angle between the empirically determined axis through the talus and the center line of the tibia is measured with a second goniometer which has

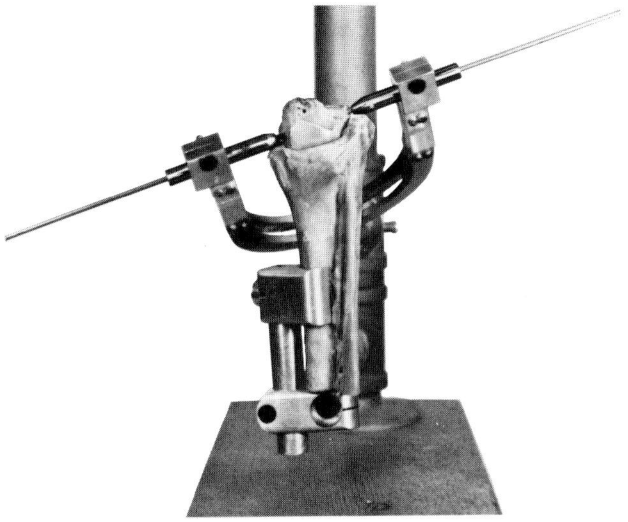

FIG. A-7. Apparatus with articulator and talus holder removed. The talus remains rigidly fixed by the 3-mm stainless steel rod held in the axis locator. Movement of the talus within the mortise is checked as it is forced to rotate about a fixed axis.

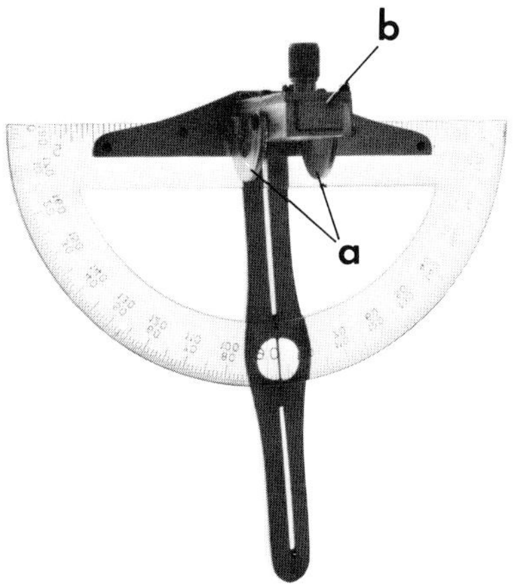

FIG. A-8. Posterior view of special goniometer. *a*, Two hemidisks fixed to movable slide. These orient the edge of the protractor to a plane which corresponds to the lateral and medial articular surfaces and ignores the variable medial elevation. *b*, Movable slide permitting hemidisks to be adjusted so as to contact bottom of anteroposterior concavity of plafond.

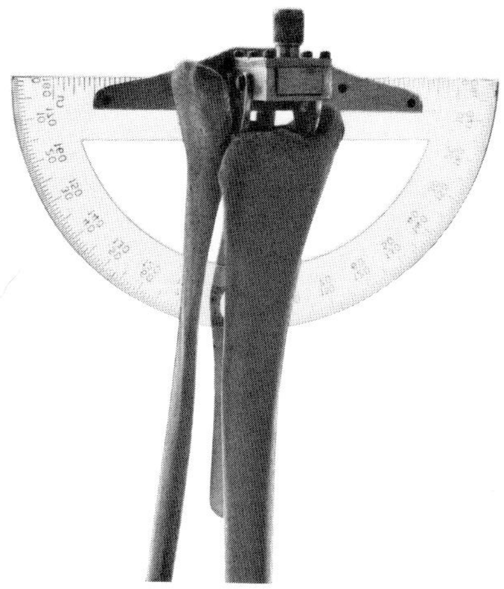

FIG. A-9. Posterior view of goniometer applied to dry bony specimen to demonstrate positioning of hemidisks within mortise.

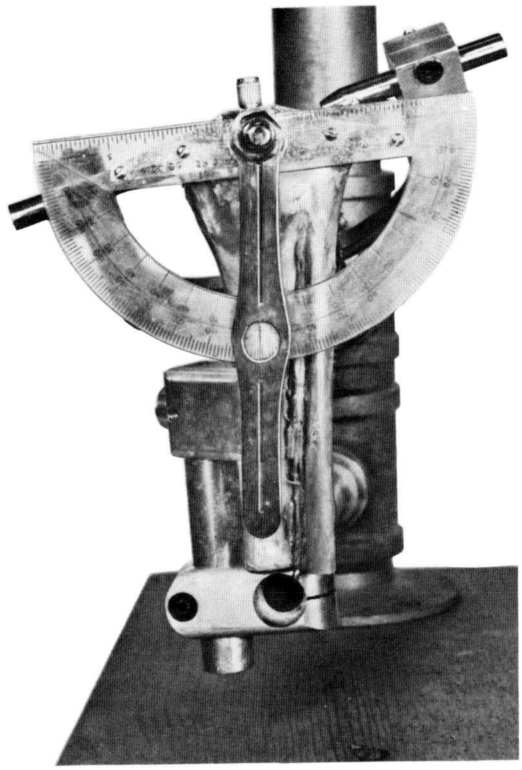

FIG. A-10. Use of special goniometer to determine angle between plafond of mortise and long axis of tibia.

curved brackets that fit over the drill guides so that it aligns itself parallel to the axis (Fig. A-11).

Step 12. The stainless steel rod (without the talus) is reinserted through the guide holes in the axis locator stirrup. Masking tape is wrapped around the periphery of the mortise and extended upward to include the stainless steel rod representing the empirically determined axis of the ankle joint. The receptacle formed by the mortise and its surrounding masking tape is filled with liquid dental stone to a height sufficient to enclose the stainless steel rod. The preparation is tapped gently to cause the dental stone to fill all crevices (Fig. A-12).

Step 13. After the dental stone has set, it is removed; it provides an accurate mold of the mortise and includes the empirically determined ankle axis. This cast is labeled and set aside for further study.

Step 14. The tibia with the fibula and the talus are removed from the clamp and replaced in preserving fluid to prevent drying while awaiting further study.

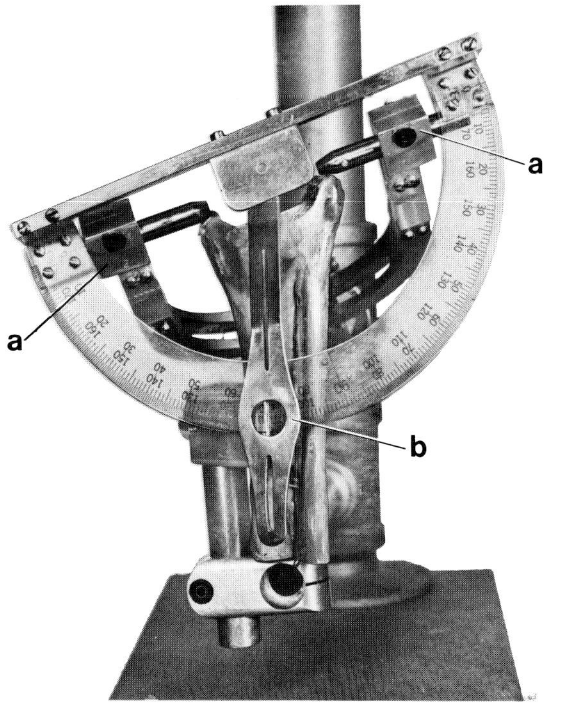

FIG. A-11. Second goniometer constructed to determine angle between empirically located axis of ankle joint and midline of tibia. *a*, Shallow stirrups located at each end of frames supporting protractor and fitting over drill guides, which correspond to empirical axis. *b*, Movable arm for measuring angle between axis and midline of tibia.

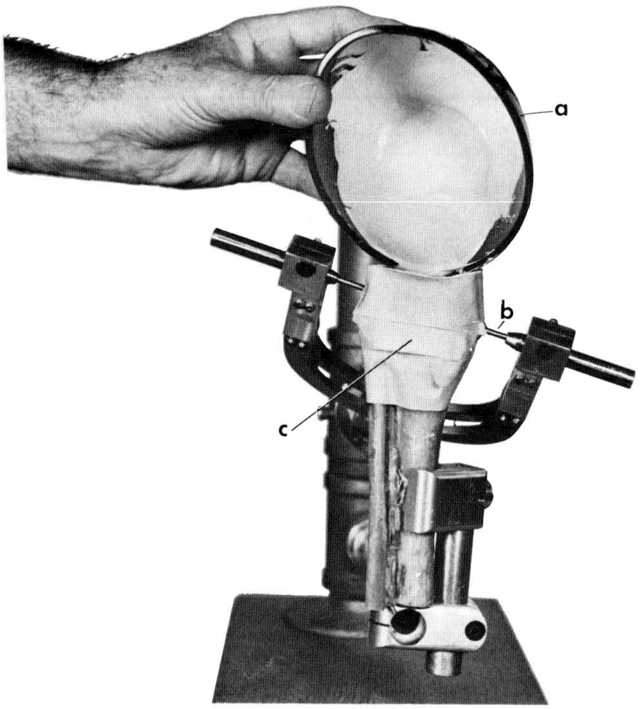

FIG. A-12. Method for taking cast of mortise. *a*, Liquid dental stone; *b*, 3-mm axis rod reinserted through drill guides to relate empirical axis to cast; *c*, receptacle of masking tape to contain dental stone.

appendix B

methods used for the measurement of trochlear widths

Method (According to Barnett and Napier, 1952) Employed to Measure the Widths of the Trochleas in Planes Always Perpendicular to the Surfaces of the Tibial Facets. A small flat stainless steel plate was rigidly fixed to one arm of a compass, in a plane at a right angle to the plane of the compass. On the other arm of the compass was an adjustable pointer (Fig. B-1). This special caliper was constructed and used in the following manner.

The flat plate was held firmly against the surface of the tibial facet and the calipers were closed until the pointer contacted the lateral (fibular) surface of the trochlea (Fig. B-2). Since the edge joining the superior surface of the trochlea and the fibular facet was always rounded, it was necessary to place the tip of the pointer on the spot which appeared to represent the superior border of the true surface of the fibular facet. When the posterior width of the trochlea was measured, the flattened triangular facet (for the inferior transverse ligament of the tibiofibular syndesmosis) was included in the width. Three dimensions were measured, one at the anterior margin, one in the approximate center, and the last at the posterior margin of the articular surface of the fibular facet. Measurements were made to the nearest millimeter and recorded. Cadaver specimens (107) were used.

Method employed to measure the widths of the trochleas and their mortises along "saw cuts." Specimens used in this study consisted of tali and the casts of their corresponding mortises, in which saw cuts had been made (see Appendix E). The length of each saw cut in the trochleas (Fig. B-3) and their corresponding casts (Fig. B-4) was measured with a pair of bow dividers. The arms of the dividers were fitted with extensions of 2-mm stainless steel rods bent and provided with small tapered nibs. The nibs held the pointers in the ends of the saw cuts as the dividers were closed to contact the articular surfaces. The measurements were taken at the superior margins of the true tibial and fibular facets. The dimensions were recorded to the nearest millimeter in 107 tali and casts of mortises. The beveled triangular area of the posterolateral aspect of the trochlea was included in the measured width.

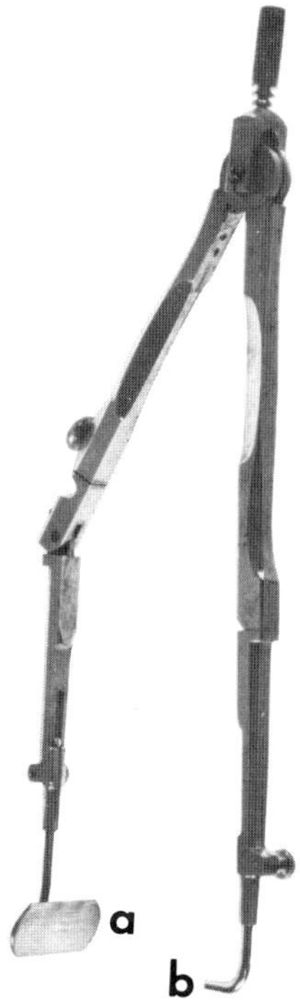

FIG. B-1. Calipers employed to measure width of trochlea at right angle to plane of tibial facet. *a*, Flat plate for surface of tibial facet; *b*, blunt pointer for fibular facet.

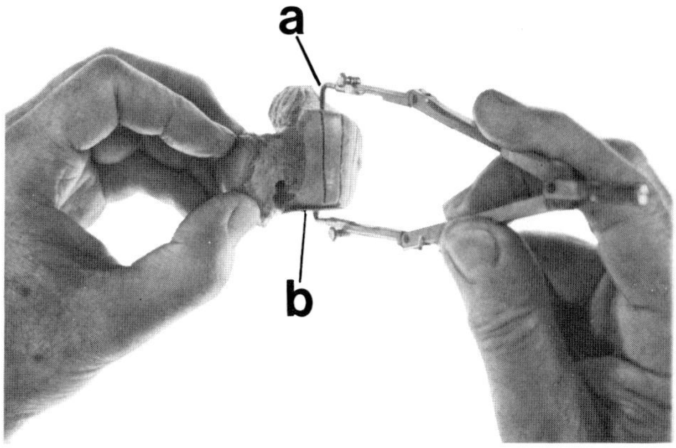

FIG. B-2. Method of employing calipers to measure width of trochlea. *a*, Pointer applied to fibular facet. *b*, flat plate applied to tibial facet.

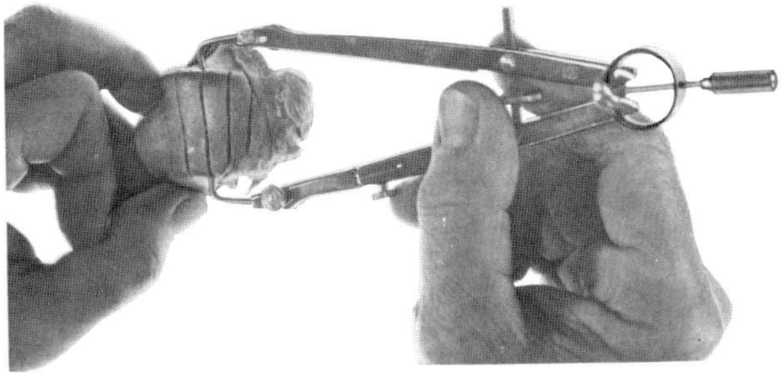

FIG. B-3. Bow dividers being used to measure width of trochlea along saw cuts in talus.

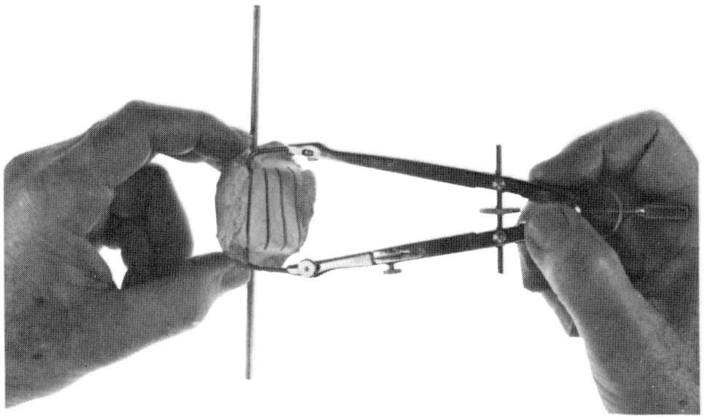

FIG. B-4. Bow dividers being used to measure width of mortise along saw cuts in cast of mortise.

appendix C

method used to measure the angles between the vertical planes of the fibular and tibial facets and the empirically located axis of the ankle joint

A special goniometer was constructed. It consisted of a plastic protractor mounted on a movable mechanical parallelogram. One arm of the mechanical parallelogram was rigidly fixed parallel to a 3-mm stainless steel rod. The longer arm of the rod was for insertion into the drill hole previously made (see Appendix A), which represented the ankle axis. The shorter arm carried a pointer. The scale was free to move with one arm of the parallelogram (Fig. C-1).

The rod was inserted through the drill hole, and the angles between the ankle axis and the tibial facet (Fig. C-2,*A*) and the ankle axis and the fibular facet (Fig. C-2,*B*) were measured. The surfaces of the tibial facets were reasonably flat. The fibular facets were curved to varying extents, requiring that a tangent be estimated by eye. The accuracy of the angular measurements on the fibular side, therefore, was not as precise as one would desire. However, repeated measurements upon the same specimen on different days and by different investigators showed the individual measurements to be within 4° of one another.

The casts of the mortises were measured in a manner similar to that used for the tali (Fig. C-3). A series of 107 cadaver tali and casts were measured in this manner. The results are given in the text.

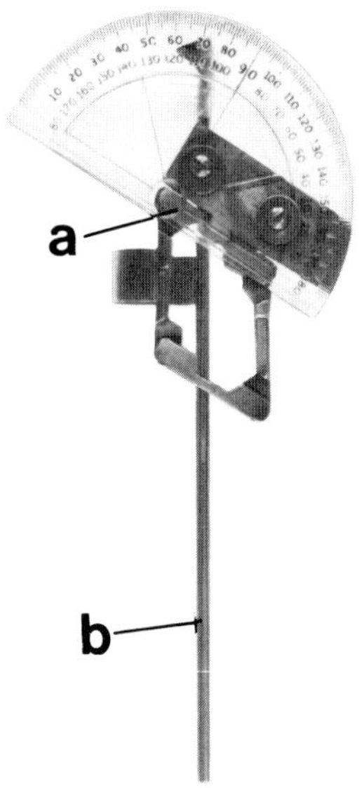

FIG. C-1. Goniometer for measuring angle between planes of tibial and fibular facets and empirically located axis of ankle joint. *a*, Movable protractor attached to one side of parallelogram; *b*, rod for insertion into drill hole in talus, which orients goniometer to ankle axis.

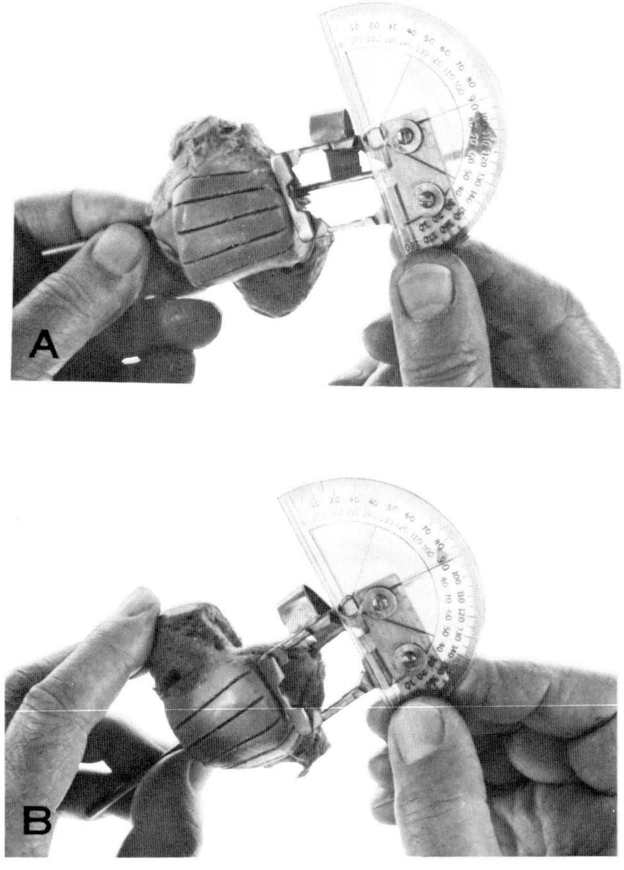

FIG. C-2. Method of measuring angles between planes of tibial and fibular facets and axis of ankle joint. *A*, Tibial facet; *B*, fibular facet.

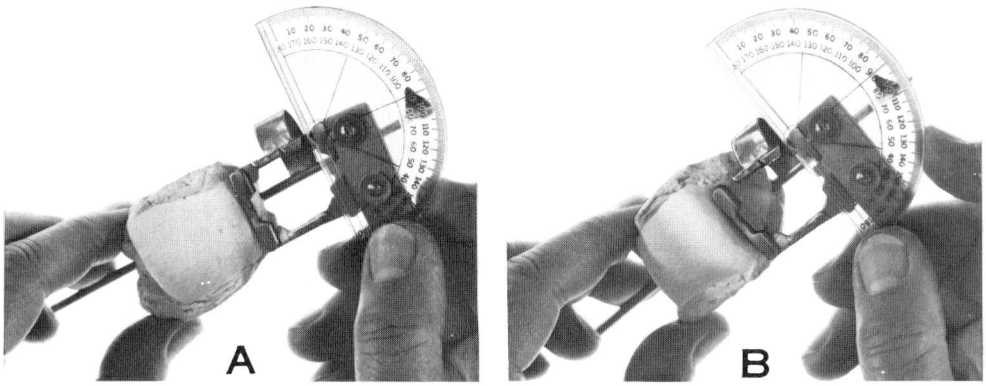

FIG. C-3. Method of measuring angles of tibial (*A*) and fibular (*B*) facets on casts of mortises.

appendix D

methods used to determine the curvatures of the superior surfaces of the trochleas and their corresponding casts

In this study of the curvature of the trochlea, three procedures and several different pieces of equipment were employed. In all 107 specimens the contourometer was used. In 59 specimens the "Formagage" was employed as a rapid check, and in a selected group of 30 specimens a visual check was added in which a modified caliper was used.

It is apparent that in studying a convex surface, all three of the techniques are readily applicable. However, in measuring the curvature of a concave surface, neither the contourometer nor the caliper could be satisfactorily used, since the data would consist in estimating the movement of a point. Therefore, casts of the mortises (see Appendix A) were employed and measured precisely, as were the tali.

The Contourometer. A special apparatus was constructed (Fig. D-1). It consisted of two metal turntables mounted on ball bearings and connected by gears and a chain. No play occurred between the turntables. In the center of one was a shaft into which a 3-mm rod could be inserted and fixed with a thumbscrew. Each talus (or cast) with its 3-mm rod representing the empirically located axis of the ankle joint (see Appendix A) was securely held to its metal axis by two collars with projecting prongs. The axial rod was mounted in the shaft of the turntable. The talus or cast could then be rotated in space about its empirically determined axis. Firmly fixed to the base of the apparatus was a vertical member which carried a movable horizontal arm. At one end of the arm was an adjustable rod carrying a tiny ball bearing (3 mm). The outer race of the bearing contacted the articular surface of the trochlea, providing smooth and relatively frictionless movement.

At the other end of the movable horizontal arm was mounted a spring-loaded ball-point pen which played against the surface of the second turntable. A card (10 × 15 cm) could be placed on the surface of the turntable and held with four microscope slide clips. The apparatus was tested for accuracy of reproduction using various irregularly shaped sections of plastic rods (see Fig. D-1).

After the specimens were mounted they were rotated through an angular range permitted by the articular surfaces. Three contours were recorded, one at the most lateral edge, one at the medial edge, and one in the approximate center. The position of each contour was marked on each talus with an indelible pencil and transferred to the cast of its corresponding mortise. This was necessary for making comparable measurements between the cadaver tali and their casts.

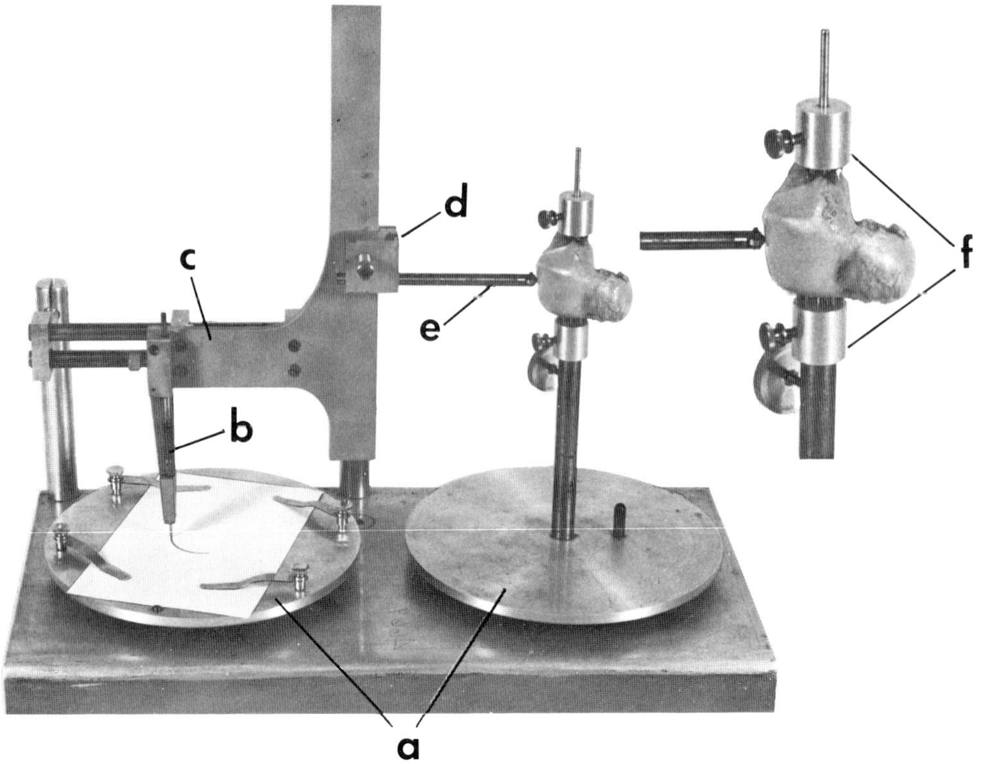

FIG. D-1. Contourometer. The *inset* shows in greater detail the method of mounting the talus (or the cast of the mortise) on the axle of one turntable and the small (3 mm) ball bearing which contacted the articular surface of the trochlea. *a*, Turntables linked together by gears and a bicycle chain within base of contourometer. *b*, Spring-loaded ball-point pen for recording curvature on data card. *c*, Horizontal slide for transmission of displacement of contour rod to ball-point pen. Constant contact of the contour rod with its ball bearing was maintained by rubber bands not visible in the photograph. *d*, Vertical slide for adjusting contour rod to desired levels on trochlea. *e*, Contour rod carrying small ball bearing. *f*, Collars for holding talus.

The data reduction was similar to that used with the Formagage and will be described below.

The Formagage. The Formagage (Penn Industries, Philadelphia, Pennsylvania) is a commercially available instrument for contouring irregular surfaces. Its use is simple and convenient and is clearly depicted in Figure D-2. When used, it was held as nearly perpendicular as possible to the 3-mm rod representing the ankle axis. After contouring of the surface of the specimen, the instrument was locked and the curvature was transferred with a sharply pointed pencil to the data cards (Fig. D-2).

The curvature of each specimen was recorded on cards with information derived from either the contourometer or the Formagage. A transparent plastic overlay was precision-engraved with circles of varying radii with 2-mm increments. The recorded arcs were matched as accurately as possible to the inscribed circles in the plastic overlay (Fig. D-3), in order to locate the arc and its center. At this center a circle was drawn with a compass; then the extent to which the recorded curvature deviated from the arc of a true circle could be readily determined.

In the complete series of 107 tali, 86 of the recorded curvatures could be fitted to an arc of a circle within 1 mm. Reproductions of typical data cards are shown in Figure D-4. In the remaining 21 tali, one or more of the recorded contour curves could not be accurately fitted to an arc of a circle. An example of one of the poorest fits is shown in Figure D-4 (lower card).

It was thought that the inability to demonstrate the curvature of the trochlea of the talus to be an arc of a true circle in 20% (21/107) of the specimens might be due to errors in the two techniques employed. Therefore, these 21 specimens and selected specimens showing good circularity were rechecked with a specially modified pair of calipers; a 3-mm rod was inserted into one arm and an adjustable pointer into the other. The rod was inserted into the drill hole of the specimen and the dividers were closed until the pointer contacted the articular surface of the trochlea (Fig. D-5). The caliper was rotated and deviations from circularity could be readily seen. This visual check confirmed the accuracy of both the contourometer and the Formagage and demonstrated the noncircularity of the 21 specimens. A review of the data

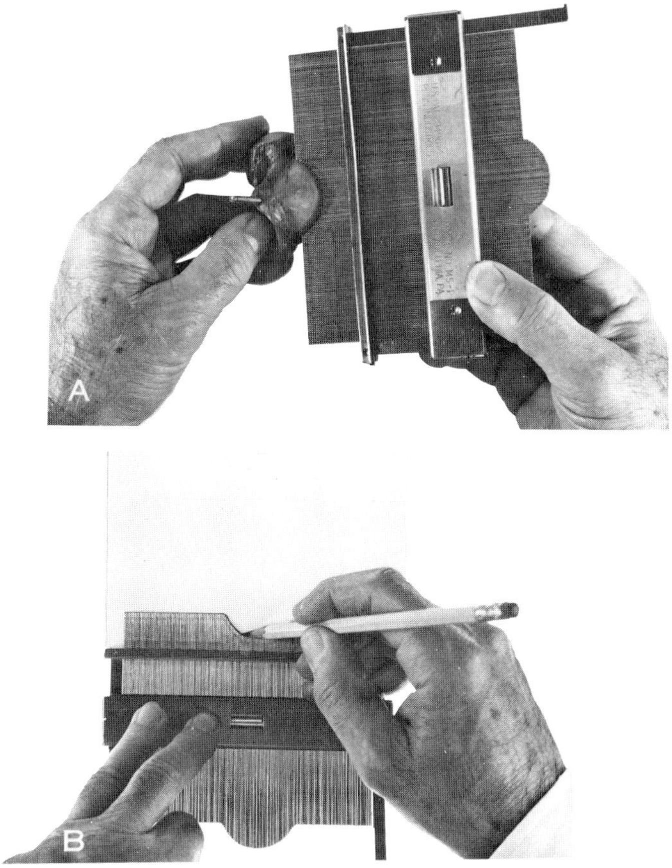

FIG. D-2. Formagage. *A*, Method of using Formagage to obtain curvature of trochlea; *B*, transference of curvature to data card after gage is locked.

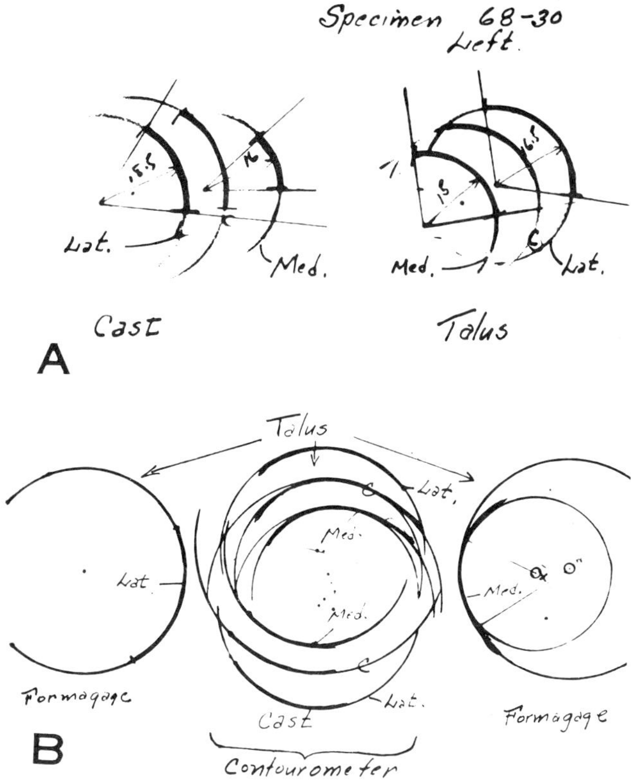

FIG. D-4. Samples of typical data cards. With use of the centers determined from the plastic overlay, arcs of circles have been drawn with a compass. Coincidence or deviations of the contours from true circularity can be readily seen. The *upper card* shows good coincidence while the *lower card* shows deviations.

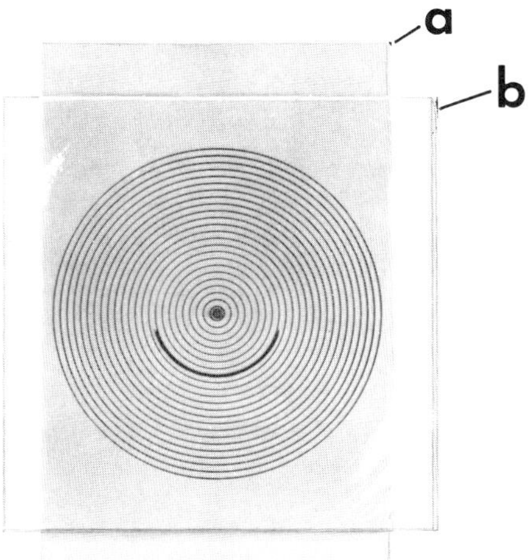

FIG. D-3. Method of determining center of arc of curvature of trochlea obtained from contourometer or Formagage. *a*, Data card on which arc of curvature has been recorded; *b*, precision-engraved plastic overlay used to determine center of recorded arcs.

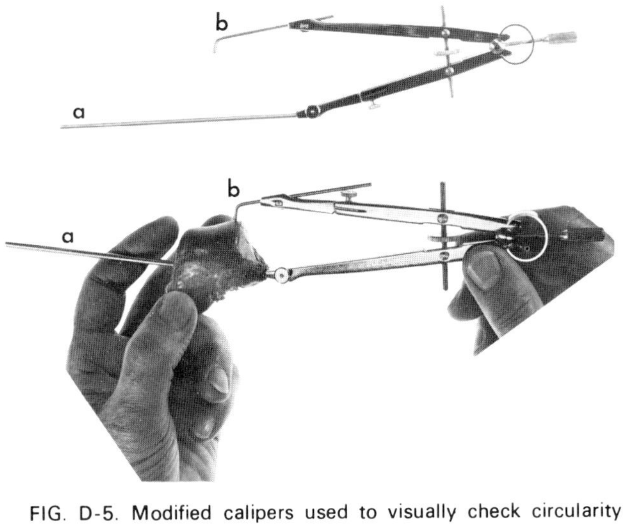

FIG. D-5. Modified calipers used to visually check circularity of trochlear surface. *a*, 3-mm rod for insertion into hole representing previously determined empirical axis. *b*, Adjustable pointer to contact articular surface of trochlea as caliper is rotated around its fixed axis running through talus.

showed that deviations from arcs of circles occurred almost exclusively on the medial side. Nineteen specimens, while demonstrating circularity on the lateral side of the trochlea, deviated from circularity on the medial side. Two specimens demonstrated noncircularity on both sides.

The data cards of the 86 tali which demonstrated good circularity of the trochlea were selected for measurement of the radii of curvature. The radii were measured from the circles inscribed on the cards and represented the medial and lateral sides. The radius of the middle contour was not measured. The arcs of circles for the casts were also available on the same data card, having been contoured at the same relative locations as their tali (Fig. D-4). Measurements were made to the nearest half-millimeter on a steel scale.

The data were tabulated and comparisons were made between the radii on the two sides of the talus and between corresponding radii on the talus and the cast of the mortise.

appendix E

method employed to visually demonstrate the conical shape of the trochlea by means of saw cuts

The use of saw cuts into the trochlea to demonstrate that they converged toward the medial side was first made on a freshly amputated undissected ankle by Close and Inman (1952). This procedure was modified and extended in an anthropometric study of 107 cadaver specimens. Several pieces of equipment were constructed to expedite the making of the saw cuts and to measure the conical angle on each talus and on the cast of its corresponding mortise.

Saw Guide (Fig. E-1). A 9-mm metallic bow was constructed which could be rotated in two planes and locked to a heavy plastic (Formica) plate. At both ends of the bow were 3-mm holes with setscrews to receive and fix the 3-mm rod representing the empirical axis of the ankle joint. Immediately above the 3-mm screw holes were slotted extensions for the blade of a hack saw. The slots were aligned so that the saw blade lay in the same vertical plane as the 3-mm rod representing the empirical axis of the ankle joint. A circular arm was attached at a right angle to the center of the bow, on which graduation marks were imprinted at 15° intervals. Through a chuck, mounted on this arm, a threaded screw pin could be inserted into the talus or the cast for fixation and graduated motion.

In use, the talus (or cast) was placed in the center of the bow. A 15-cm rod, 3 mm in diameter, was inserted through the bow and the drill hole in the talus. The specimen was fixed by the threaded pin. The talus was rotated until either the posterior or anterior edge of the articular surface of the trochlea lay in the vertical plane of the saw blade. All movable parts were rigidly fixed with thumbscrews. With a saw, a cut approximately 6 mm deep was made into the trochlea. The saw blade was elevated and the talus was rotated 15° about its empirical axis. The specimen was again rigidly clamped and another saw cut was made. This procedure was repeated until saw cuts had been made over the entire trochlear surface. Usually, there were four to six cuts per specimen (Fig. E-2). In no specimens were the saw cuts parallel; they converged toward the medial side of the talus or cast.

Measurement of the Conical Angle. To determine the angle of convergence of the saw cuts and to calculate the average conical angle of each trochlea and cast, a special goniometer was constructed (Fig. E-3). This consisted of a wooden base 51 cm long, provided with two 7.6-cm brass pillars 46 cm apart. A 3-mm rod passed through holes in each pillar and supported the talus by passing through the drill hole of the ankle axis. A 1-mm stainless steel pin was forcibly pushed into one of the saw cuts. Because the center of the trochlea exhibited a slight concavity of varying depth, the pin was made flush with the medial and lateral surfaces only and the central concavity was ignored. The talus was rotated until the pin in the saw cut lay in the same horizontal plane as the rod representing the ankle axis. In most of the specimens the saw cut pin crossed this rod at varying distances and angles on the medial side of the specimen.

A plastic protractor was mounted horizontally in such a way that it could be slid toward or away from the specimen until the center of the protractor overlay the point of intersection of the axis rod and the pin in the saw cuts. The angle between rod and pin was recorded to the nearest estimated degree.

The procedure was repeated for each saw cut. Because of various factors, the differences between individual measurements on each saw cut differed from 1 to 5°, so that there were inaccuracies of this magnitude inherent in the method. In the hope that the variations were randomly distributed, the four to six measurements were averaged for each specimen.

The conical angle of the trochlea was calculated for each specimen by multiplying the average angle of convergence of the saw cuts by two.

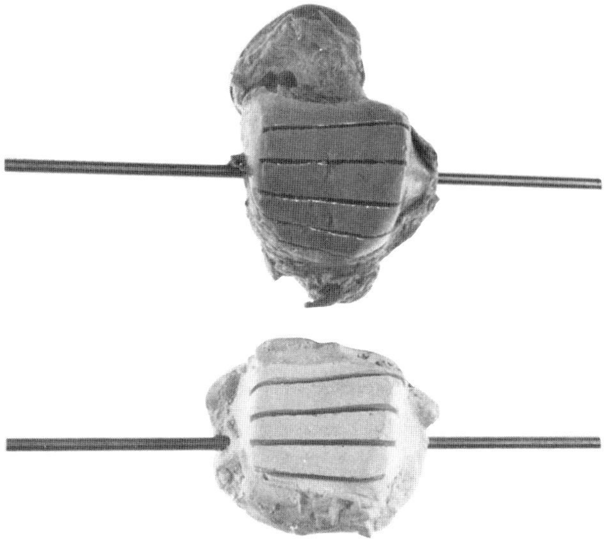

FIG. E-2. Typical talus and cast of its mortise after saw cuts have been made.

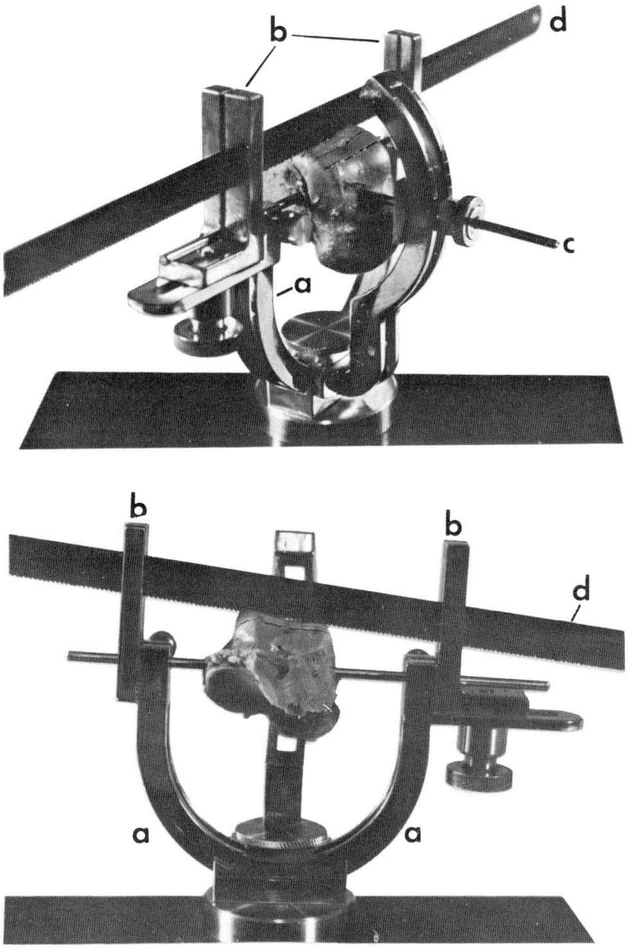

FIG. E-1. Saw guide. *a*, Adjustable metal bow supporting talus on 3-mm rod that represents empirical axis; *b*, slotted saw guides; *c*, screw pin inserted into nonarticular part of talus and held in chuck, which can be moved along circular track to turn and fix talus in various degrees of rotation; *d*, saw blade from which frame has been removed.

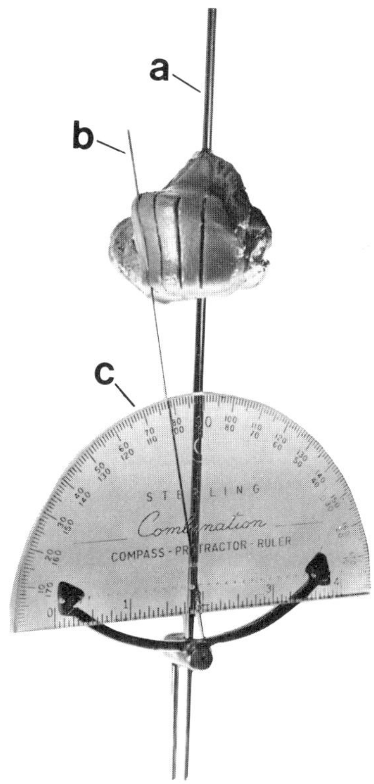

FIG. E-3. Goniometer employed to measure angle of convergence of saw cuts. *a*, 3-mm stainless steel rod on which talus and protractor are mounted; *b*, stiff stainless steel Kirschner wire pressed into saw cut; *c*, protractor, which is slid along axis rod until its center lies over point of intersection of Kirschner wire and 3-mm axis rod.

appendix F

method of locating the subtalar axis, measuring the range of motion about it, and analyzing the "screwlike" motion of the talus on the calcaneus

Location of the Subtalar Axis (Fig. F-1). The calcaneus is firmly held in a clamp (*a*) rigidly fixed to a pipe frame.

The talus is articulated on the calcaneus. Sharp pointers (as employed in Appendix A) are inserted into the stirrup (*b*). The stirrup is moved by means of a jointed support until the talar pointer locates the point of minimal motion on the talus as it is moved through its full range while the articular surfaces are manually held in contact. The talar pointer is driven into the bone sufficiently to mark the point of minimal motion. The process is then reversed, the talus is clamped, and the calcaneus is moved on the talus. The point of minimal motion on the calcaneus is located. The stirrup is adjusted until the two pointers, when gently pressed into the bone, align the two points of minimal motion. Accuracy of location of the functional axis is checked by moving the joint through its range of motion and observing any restriction of motion or movement of the pointers, as well as preservation of contact of the articular surfaces.

The stirrup is locked and the pointers are replaced with drill guides. The stirrup now acts as a jig for the drill. A 3-mm drill is passed through both bones and replaced with a 3-mm stainless steel rod (see Fig. F-1). The two bones are removed from the apparatus and the accuracy of placement of the axis is checked. If restriction of motion or separation of articular surfaces has occurred, the process of axis location is repeated.

All tali and calcanei were left articulated, with their 3-mm stainless steel axes in place, and returned to containers with preservative fluid until used for further study.

Series I (47 Specimens). Since only ranges of motion were being considered in this series, the method consisted of clamping the calcaneus and mounting a protractor perpendicular to the stainless steel rod which constituted the functional axis. A flexible pointer was drilled into the fixed calcaneus. Rotation of the talus with its protractor revealed the range of motion.

Two sets of measurements were made on each specimen. The first set of measurements was made with capsular and ligamentous structures intact and the second, with all ligamentous restraints removed.

Series II. The intent of this study on cadaver tali and calcanei was to reinvestigate the screwlike motion of the talus on the calcaneus. Such action had been reported in the literature. Two separate series of measurements were made. The first consisted of an investigation of the curvature of the posterior facet of the calcaneus, in an attempt to collect data from which a helix angle could be calculated. The second was a series of direct measurements on the absolute linear displacement of the talus along its empirically determined axis during rotation of the talus on the calcaneus.

In both studies the basic apparatus consisted of a turntable with a protruding axle. The axle had been drilled to receive the 3-mm stainless steel rod. The turntable had been calibrated for rotation to 1°. To an outrigger was fixed a dial gage calibrated to 0.025 mm (Fig. F-2).

For the studies of the curvature of the posterior facet of the calcaneus the talus was removed and the calcaneus was rigidly mounted on the turntable. The arm carrying the dial gage was adjusted to contact the articular surface and to record deflections over the entire extent of the articular surface as the turntable rotated the calcaneus. The articular surface was contoured at 5 and 10 mm from the center of the empirical axis. Recordings from the dial gage were made for every 10° of rotation (Fig. F-3).

The curves of the plotted values showed such individual variations that it was felt of interest to present the actual data on 10 of the 49 specimens studied. These were selected as representative of typical patterns and are reproduced in Figures F-4 through F-7.

To measure the absolute linear displacement of the talus along the empirical axis, the turntable was locked and a protractor was fixed to the shaft to record rotations. The talus was articulated upon the

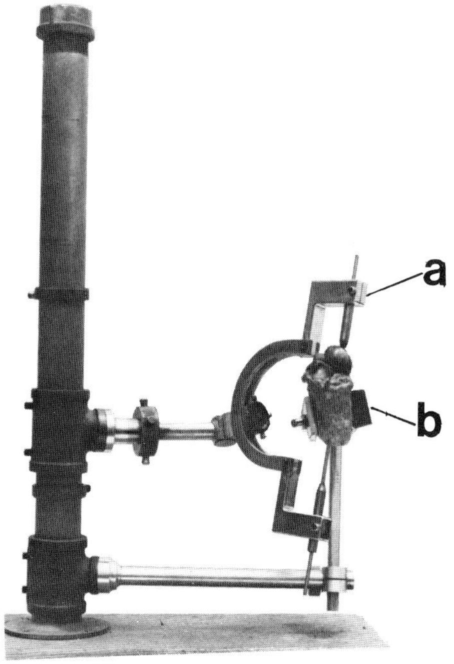

FIG. F-1. Apparatus used to determine axis of subtalar joint. *a*, Adjustable stirrup holding same pointers and drill guides as were employed for studies described in Appendix A; *b*, clamp to secure calcaneus (or talus).

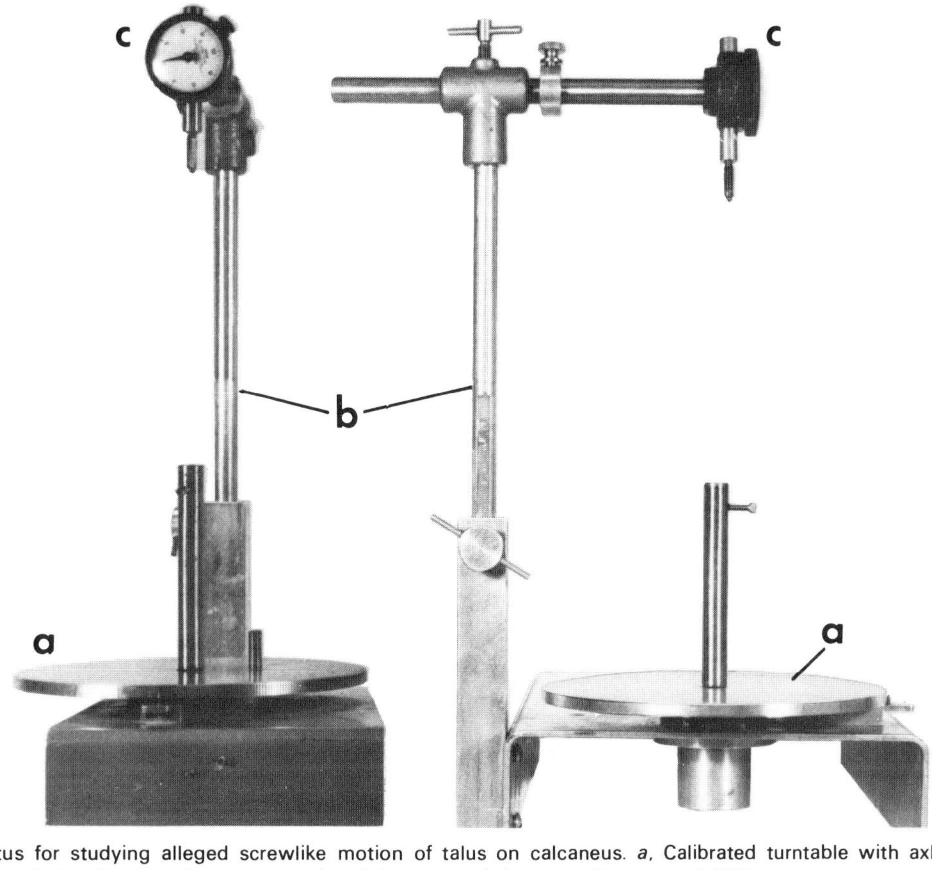

FIG. F-2. Apparatus for studying alleged screwlike motion of talus on calcaneus. *a*, Calibrated turntable with axle drilled to accept 3-mm stainless steel rod; *b*, adjustable frame supporting dial gage; *c*, dial gage calibrated to 0.025 mm.

calcaneus. The 3-mm rod representing the empirical axis was extended into the talus but only sufficiently far to assure that rotation of the talus occurred around it. The upper end of the rod was left approximately 5 mm short of protruding from the neck of the talus. To provide a flat surface perpendicular to the arm of the dial gage, a flat-headed copper rivet was gently pushed into the drill hole left unoccupied by the rod. The shank of the rivet was not long enough to contact the axial rod, and its fit in the drill hole was sufficiently snug to force it to follow all motions of the talus. To record the amount of rotation of the talus upon the fixed calcaneus a pointer was inserted in the talus. The stem of the dial gage was lowered to contact the head of the rivet, the talus was rotated, and recordings from the dial gage for every 10° of rotation were made (Fig. F-8).

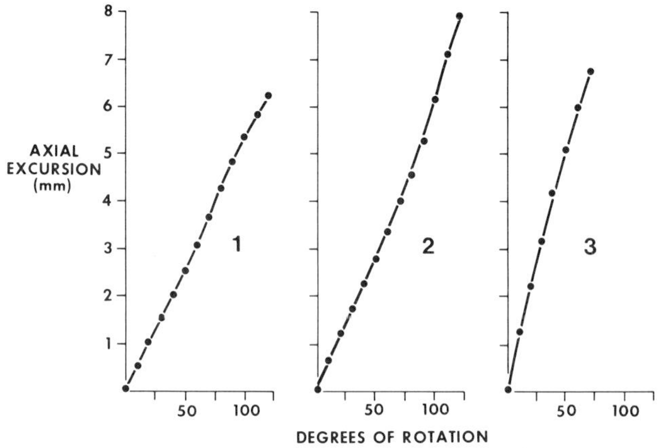

FIG. F-4. Plotted data on three specimens which are representative of a group constituting over half of specimens studied. Note that the loci may be fitted with a straight line and that while the slopes of the curves differ they suggest a pure screwlike behavior of the subtalar joint.

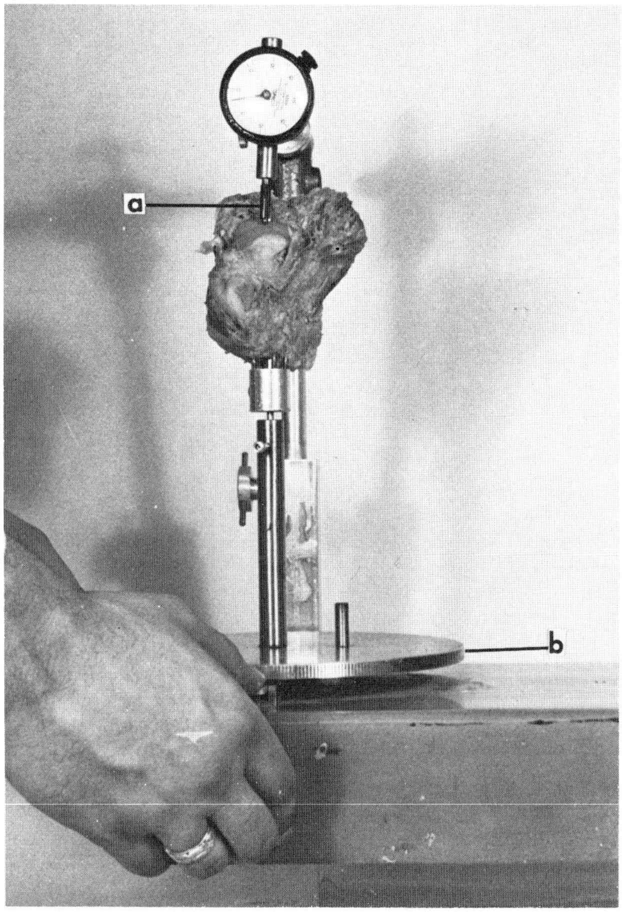

FIG. F-3. Method of studying curvature of posterior facet of calcaneus. *a*, Stem of dial gage contacting articular surface of posterior facet of calcaneus at measured distance (5 or 10 mm) from center of axis; *b*, calibrated turntable. Recordings from the dial gage were made at every 10° of rotation of the turntable.

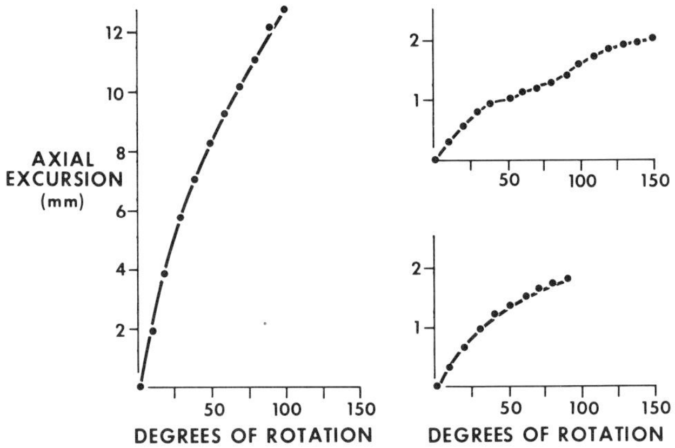

FIG. F-5. Curves revealing progressive linear displacement. The increments are not constant, however, and therefore indicate that the joint is not behaving as a true screw.

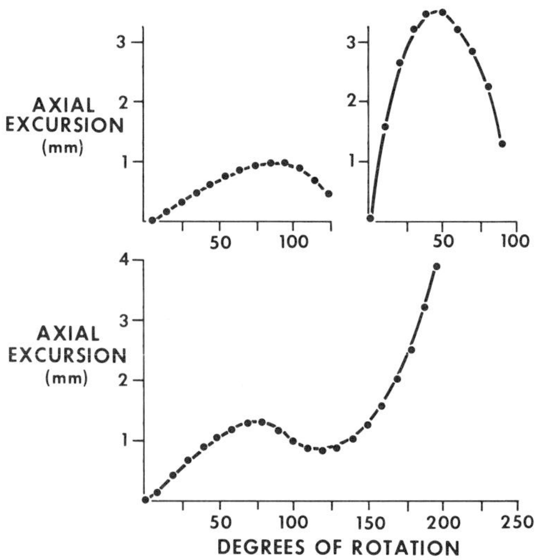

FIG. F-6. Curves revealing reversal in linear displacements, indicating divergence from true screwlike behavior.

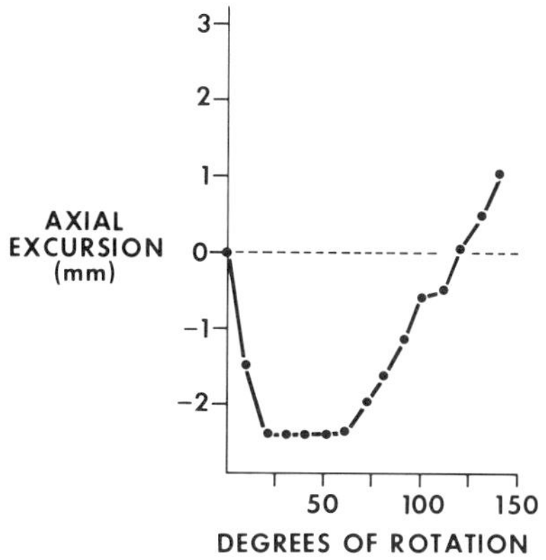

FIG. F-7. Curve representing findings in nine specimens. The initial displacement is negative, indicating a left-handed screw. There is a reversal to a right-handed screw at the termination of rotation, resulting in a total linear displacement of only 1 mm.

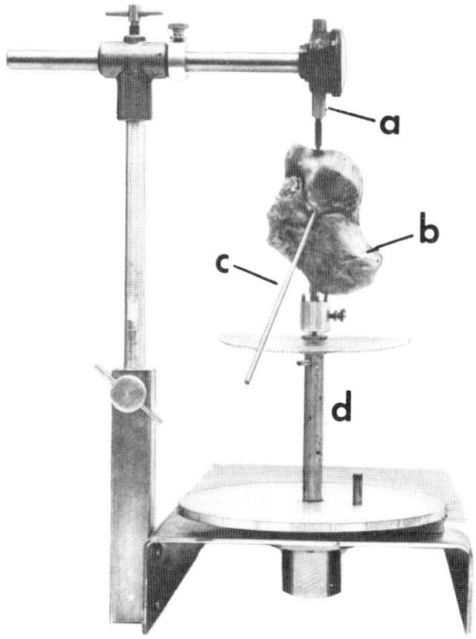

FIG. F-8. Apparatus to measure linear displacement of talus along axis of subtalar joint, with rotation of talus upon calcaneus. *a*, Stem of dial gage resting upon flat head of rivet which has been inserted into axis hole in talus; *b*, calcaneus rigidly fixed to axle of turntable; *c*, rod inserted into talus to rotate it upon fixed calcaneus, with amount of rotation indicated on protractor; *d*, turntable locked in position with protractor rigidly mounted on axle.

appendix G

method of stressing the ankle joint to determine the amount of talar tilt

The literature contains several articles which report varying amounts of talar tilt when the ankle is stressed by forceful inversion of the foot. While variations between individuals have been amply demonstrated, the possible differences in the amounts of talar tilt in a single individual when the ankle is stressed in varying degrees of plantar flexion and dorsiflexion have not been adequately investigated. We therefore studied 50 randomly selected young and middle-aged men and women who denied ever having had any type of injury to their ankles. Both right and left ankles were stressed.

To control the position of the leg and foot and to apply a constant inverting force, a special device was constructed (Fig. G-1). It consisted of a padded metal trough which supported the subject's leg and was fixed to a heavy steel base. A 20-cm metal turntable, mounted on ball bearings, was carried on a movable slide. The turntable supported two vertical members, between which was mounted a plywood tilt table. On the tilt table was fixed a removable plastic heel cup. Several sizes of heel cups were available for different individuals, and for each measurement one was selected that provided a snug fit between heel and cup. The tilt table could be rotated about a transverse axis to provide dorsiflexion and plantar flexion and could be locked in a fixed position with thumbscrews. The angle of the tilt table could be determined by a goniometer affixed to its transverse axis.

The testing procedure consisted of the following steps.

Step 1. A plastic heel cup was selected that snugly fitted the subject's heel.

Step 2. The subject was placed supine on the x-ray table. The hip and knee were flexed to relax the gastrocnemius. The leg was then placed in the padded

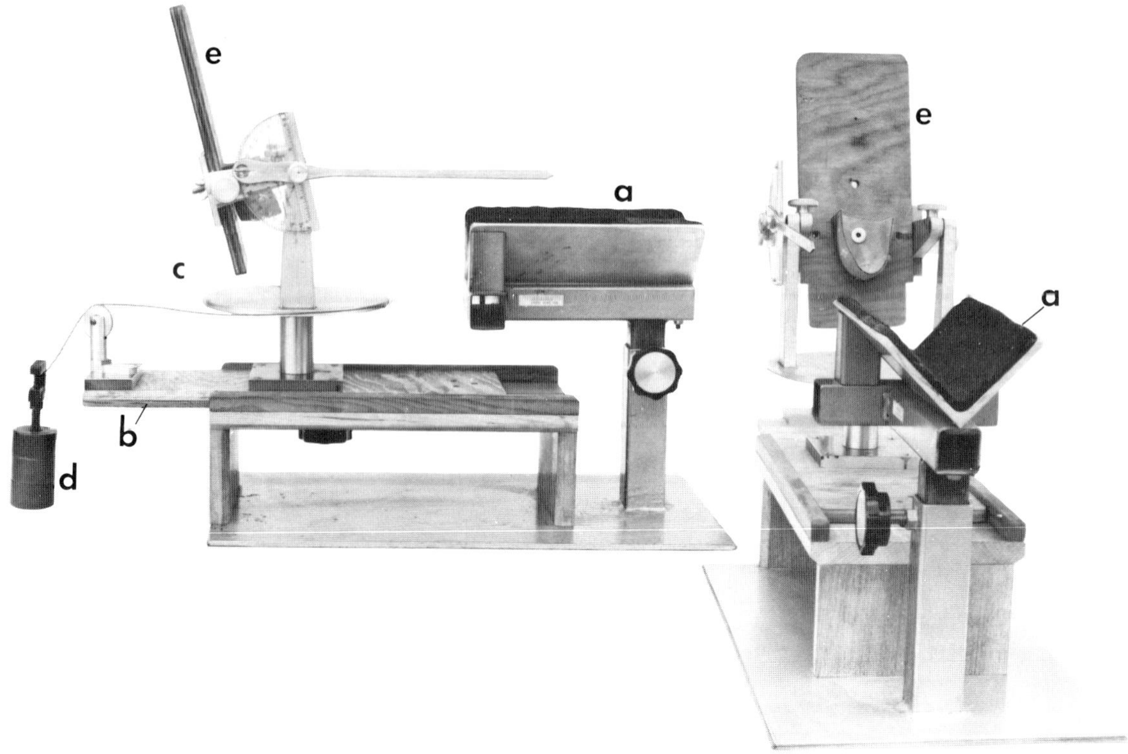

FIG. G-1. Apparatus for subjecting ankles to constant inversion stresses. *a*, Trough to support and fix leg. The trough is vertically adjustable. *b*, Slide, carrying tilt table and turntable, which may be moved horizontally to adapt to various lengths of legs. *c*, Metal turntable, 20 cm in diameter, mounted on ball bearings, which transmits torque to tilt table. *d*, 4.5-kg weight, connected by flexible cable to turntable, which when suspended exerts a constant moment of 4.4 newton meters. *e*, Adjustable tilt table to which is attached a goniometer to measure amount of plantar flexion and dorsiflexion of ankle. An appropriate size of plastic heel cup is attached to the tilt table to hold the heel securely.

metal trough and securely strapped. The ankle and foot extended beyond the trough (Fig. G-2).

Step 3. The slide supporting the turntable was adjusted so that the axis of rotation of the turntable passed through the ankle joint. The heel cup was moved on the tilt table until the horizontal axis of the tilt table was approximately parallel to a line through the tips of the malleoli.

Step 4. The forefoot was firmly fixed to the surface of the tilt table with straps. The tilt table was rotated to achieve maximal dorsiflexion and secured. The angle between the tilt table and the long axis of the leg was measured with the goniometer and recorded.

Step 5. An inversion force of 4.4 newton meters was applied to the turntable through a cord which ran around the grooved edge of the turntable, passed over a pulley, and supported a 4.5-kg weight (Fig. G-3).

Step 6. A cardboard film holder was placed on the turntable and an x-ray of the ankle was obtained with the tube 76 cm from the film holder.

Step 7. X-rays were taken of each subject with the ankle in a neutral position (90°) and in maximal plantar flexion and dorsiflexion. The degrees of plantar flexion and dorsiflexion were recorded.

Step 8. The angle of talar tilt was measured on each x-ray of each subject and was recorded.

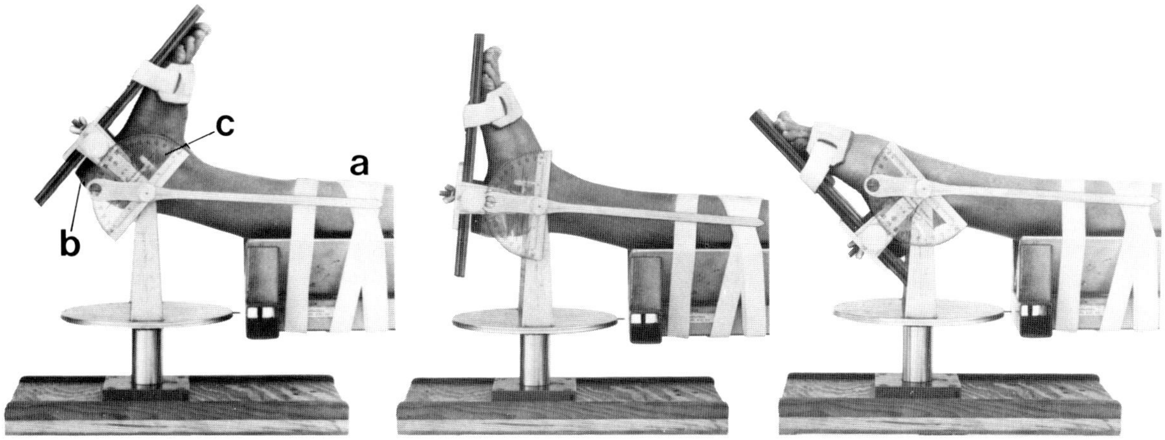

FIG. G-2. Prestressing preparation of subject in apparatus. *a*, Leg securely strapped into metal trough; *b*, heel of subject in snugly fitting plastic heel cup, with forefoot strapped to tilt table; *c*, goniometer measuring amount of plantar flexion and dorsiflexion of ankle.

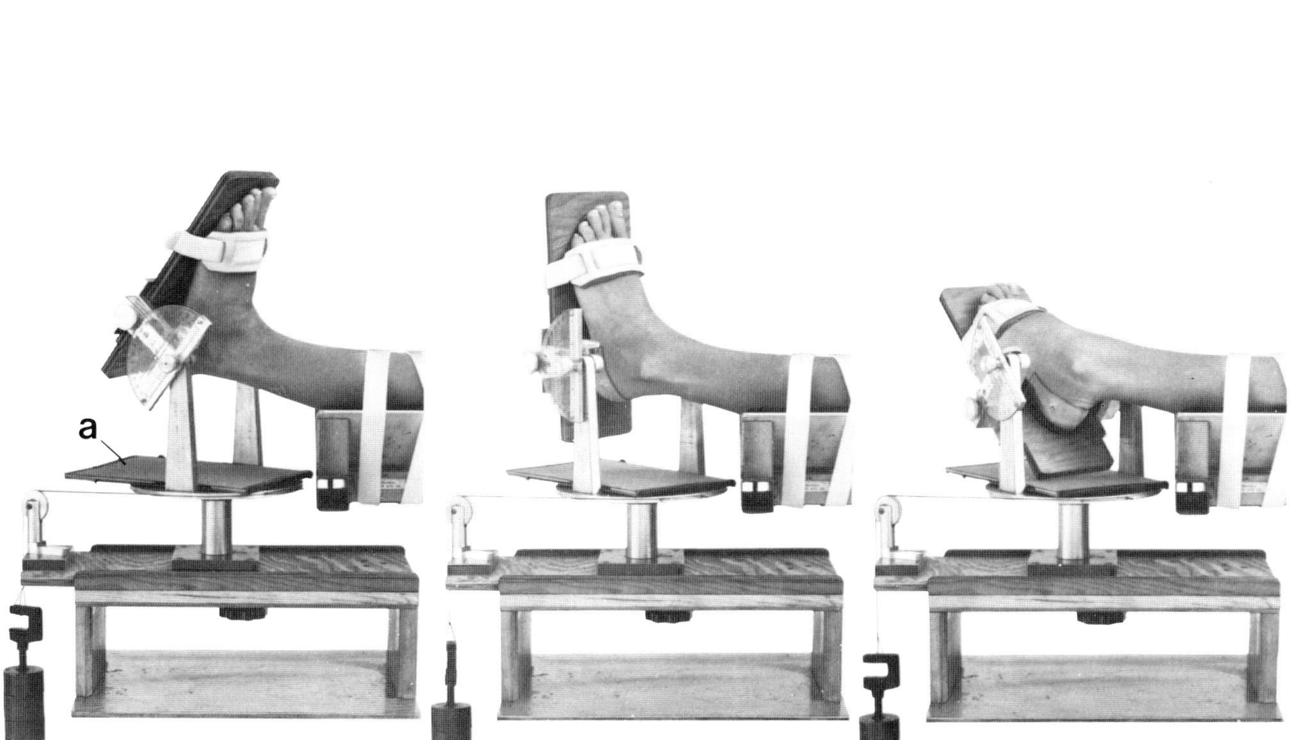

FIG. G-3. Ankle being subjected to constant inverting stress in various degrees of plantar flexion and dorsiflexion after all adjustments have been made and all parts of apparatus locked in position. *a*, Cardboard film holder placed on turntable. The x-ray tube is located at a standard 76 cm above the film.

appendix H

method of determining the angles between the axis of the subtalar joint and the calcaneofibular ligament and between the anterior talofibular and calcaneofibular ligaments

In 50 cadaver specimens all soft tissues were removed except the collateral ligaments of the ankle, which were carefully preserved. Most specimens were soaked in water for several days to make them more pliable. The subtalar axis was determined and a 3-mm stainless steel rod was inserted as outlined in Appendix F. A 1-mm Kirschner wire was threaded through the calcaneofibular ligament parallel to the direction of its fibers. A similar, but shorter, 1-mm Kirschner wire was inserted through the fibers of the anterior talofibular ligament and permitted to extend laterally (Fig. H-1).

The Angle Between the Calcaneofibular Ligament and the Axis of the Subtalar Joint. The tibia was firmly held in a clamp and fixed to a support stand by an adjustable holder. With a slight adjustment of the specimen, the rod and wire were made to lie in the same vertical plane (Fig. H-2). The angle between the two, as measured in this plane, was felt to represent the true angle of divergence between the rod and the wire.

To measure the angle between the rod and the wire a goniometer held in a horizontal plane on a separate stand was moved over the specimen and adjusted to measure the angle (Fig. H-3) in three positions of the subtalar joint: full inversion of the calcaneus, the approximate midposition, and full eversion of the calcaneus. The angular change between the rod and the wire was recorded in three positions in 50 specimens. In all specimens, in the midposition of the subtalar joint the direction of the fibers of the calcaneofibular ligament paralleled the axis of the subtalar joint surprisingly closely. The maximal deviation of about 10° from true parallelism in a few specimens could be due to errors in the location of the axis rod and in the insertion of the wire into the calcaneofibular ligament, failure to select the true midposition of the joint, and sloppy positioning of the goniometer. The average angle between the rod and the wire in the midposition of the subtalar joint was 0° ± 8°. When the leg and foot were visualized in the anatomic standing position, *i.e.*, foot flat and leg vertical as customarily depicted in textbooks, a positive value of the angle indicated that the direction of the fibers of the calcaneofibular ligament was slightly more vertical than the axis of the subtalar joint. A negative value indicated that the fibers of the calcaneofibular ligament were slightly more horizon-

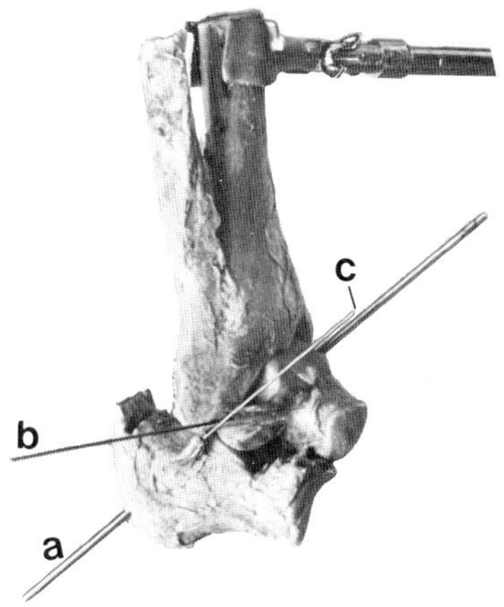

FIG. H-1. Oblique view of typical specimen. *a*, Rod inserted through talus and calcaneus in position of empirically located axis of subtalar joint; *b*, Kirschner wire inserted into anterior talofibular ligament paralleling its fibers; *c*, Kirschner wire inserted into calcaneofibular ligament paralleling its fibers.

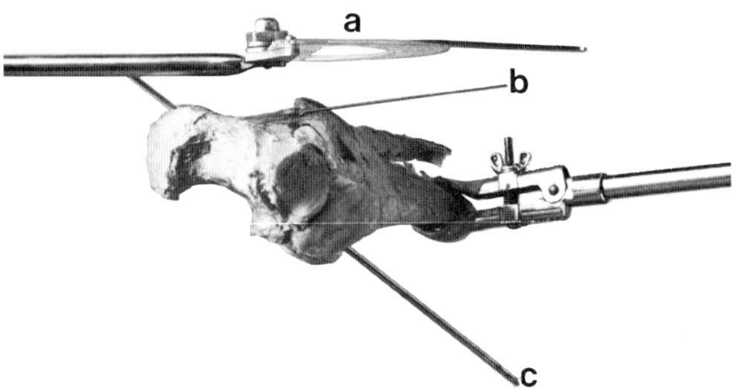

FIG. H-2. Specimen oriented so that axis rod and Kirschner wire in calcaneofibular ligament lie in same vertical plane. The goniometer has been moved over the specimen. *a*, Goniometer; *b*, Kirschner wire; *c*, axis rod.

tal than the axis of the subtalar joint. When the calcaneus was maximally inverted or everted around the subtalar axis, the degree of parallelism between the axis rod and the wire (representing the calcaneofibular ligament) was slightly decreased. With maximal inversion and eversion the direction of the fibers deviated from true parallelism by a maximal value of 19° and a minimal value of 2°. The average deviation was 14° ± 9°. The differences in the extent of deviation from parallelism with inversion and eversion of the calcaneus seem to be due to variations, in individual specimens, between the location of the calcaneal attachment of the ligament and the position of the axis rod as it emerged on the lateral side of the calcaneus. In those specimens in which the calcaneal attachment was closest to the exit of the axis rod on the lateral side of the calcaneus, there was less deviation from parallelism with inversion and eversion of the calcaneus. In all specimens, however, the ligament in no way limited the full range of movement in the subtalar joint and in no position was the ligament unduly taut or lax.

The Angle as Projected onto the Transverse Plane. When the positions of the rod representing the axis of the subtalar joint and the Kirschner wire through the calcaneofibular ligament are viewed in a horizontal plane (Fig. H-4), it will be readily seen that they intersect posteriorly and diverge anteriorly. The reason for this arrangement is obviously the necessity for the two bony attachments of the ligament to lie close to the functional axis of the ankle at its proximal end and to the functional axis of the subtalar joint at its distal end. This requires that the ligament extend from the tip of the lateral malleolus to the lateral side of the calcaneus. To fully understand the functional behavior of the ligament during movement of both ankle and subtalar joints it was felt necessary to establish the amount of divergence and the degree of individual variation. Therefore the following measurements were made on 50 cadaver specimens. Utilizing the same holding apparatus, the specimen was rotated so that the ligament and subtalar axis lay in the horizontal plane. With the goniometer mounted in a horizontal plane above the specimen, the angle between the axis rod and the Kirschner wire was measured (Fig. H-4). The average angle of divergence was 31° ± 6° with a maximal value of 43° and a minimal value of 19°.

The Angle Between the Anterior Talofibular and Calcaneofibular Ligaments. Since it has been shown that the axis of the subtalar joint varies in its inclination and since the calcaneofibular ligament has been demonstrated to closely parallel the axis when projected onto the sagittal plane, it appeared likely that the angle between the anterior talofibular and the calcaneofibular ligaments would show individual variations. The directions of the fibers of the two ligaments, however, are quite different, with the talofibular ligament coursing almost transversely and the calcaneofibular ligament running anteriorly and laterally.

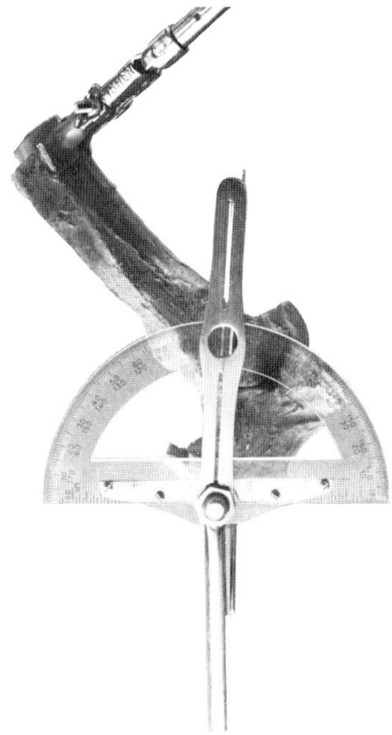

FIG. H-3. Top view showing goniometer and underlying specimen. The goniometer is moved until the center overlies the point of intersection of the rod and the wire. The angle between the rod and the wire is measured as the subtalar joint is moved through its full range.

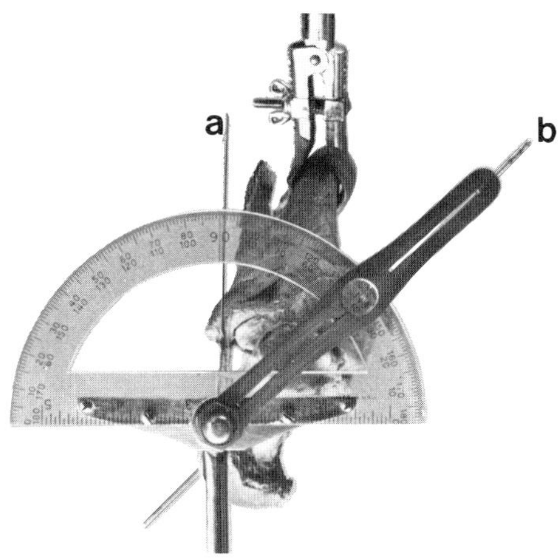

FIG. H-4. Specimen viewed from below and oriented so that axis rod and Kirschner wire lie in same horizontal plane. The divergence of the axis rod from the wire is measured with the goniometer. *a*, Kirschner wire in calcaneofibular ligament; *b*, axis rod.

The selection of a plane upon which to project and measure the angle between the two ligaments became a problem. Two planes were selected and the angle was measured in both.

The first plane was established by orienting the specimen so that the two Kirschner wires (one in the anterior talofibular ligament and the other in the calcaneofibular ligament) lay in the same horizontal plane. The goniometer, held horizontally on its own support stand, was moved over the specimen and the projected angle between the Kirschner wires in the two ligaments was measured in the midposition of the subtalar joint and in maximal inversion and eversion of the calcaneus on the talus (Fig. H-5). The average angle between the anterior talofibular ligament and the calcaneofibular ligament measured in the midposition of the subtalar joint was 105° ± 24°. A minimal value of 75° was recorded in one specimen and a maximal value of 139° in another. With inversion and eversion of the calcaneus the angle changed a varying amount in every specimen. On the average the angle decreased to 93° ± 31° on inversion and increased to 113° ± 32° on eversion. No significant differences were found between the right and left sides.

The second plane selected was one that was perpendicular to the empirical axis of the ankle joint. The specimen was rotated until the 3-mm rod representing the empirical axis of the ankle joint was vertical. The angle between the wires was measured in the same manner as above. The angle measured in this plane differed from the angle measured in the sagittal plane in most specimens. It was less in 26, greater in 13, and the same in 11 specimens. The average angle was 106° ± 24°, with a range between 86 and 128°. It was surprising to find that the average values of the angles taken in the two different planes were so comparable. Furthermore, inversion and eversion of the calcaneus produced the same change in the angle. Inversion decreased the angle to 99° ± 25° and eversion increased the angle to 111° ± 26°.

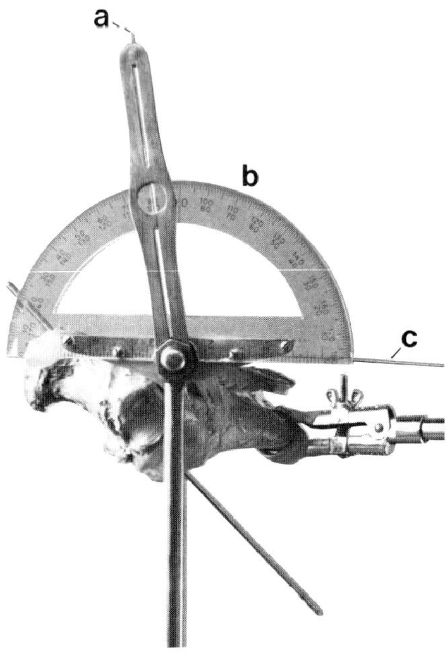

FIG. H-5. Specimen oriented by eye so that Kirschner wires inserted into calcaneofibular and anterior talofibular ligaments lie in same horizontal plane. The goniometer has been adjusted so that one wire parallels the base of the goniometer and the other wire parallels the movable arm. *a*, Wire in anterior talofibular ligament; *b*, goniometer; *c*, wire in calcaneofibular ligament.

appendix I

x-ray studies of the isolated talus and calcaneus

Fifty matched pairs of tali and calcanei were taken at random from the loan collections of prepared skeletons issued to students in gross anatomy. A 7X binocular microscope, mounted on a flexible horizontal arm which in turn could be adjusted for height on a heavy stand, was the only piece of precision equipment used. A crosshair was placed in the diaphragm of the left ocular for the fine determination of the axis of rotation in the specimens. The device for holding the talus and calcaneus was made up from odd bits of standard laboratory equipment (Figs. I-1 and I-2) (a V-jawed extension clamp, a perpendicular-jaw clamp holder, and a clamp extension bar); a small portable bench vise was used to anchor the specimen clamp firmly to the table (this was important, for during axis

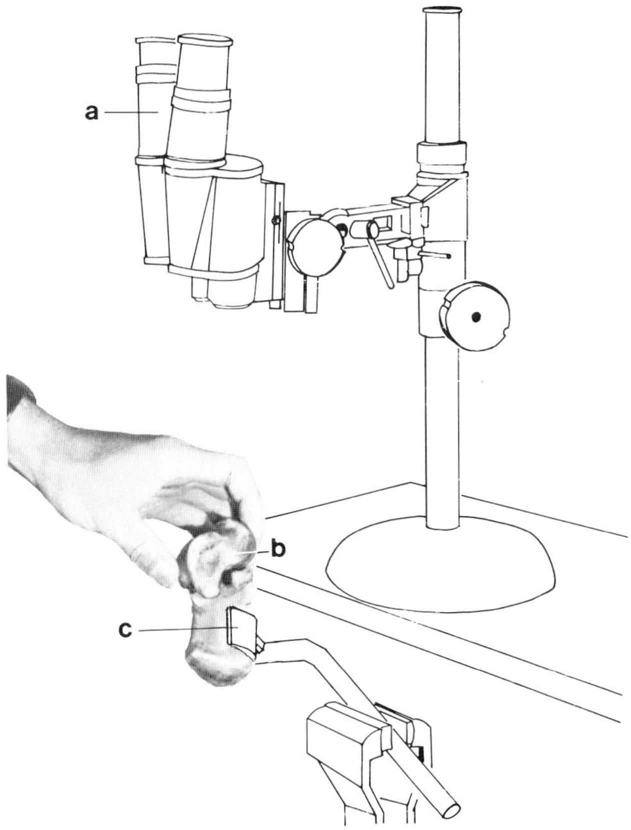

FIG. I-1. Technique for locating axis of subtalar joint in dried bony specimen. *a*, Binocular microscope, in which crosshairs are adjusted to determine point of minimal motion. This point is marked on the talus. *b*, Talus articulated on calcaneus and rotated by hand. *c*, Clamp holding calcaneus firmly.

determinations, the carefully regulated rotation of the joints could be achieved only if there was a minimum of extraneous movements and vibrations). The clamp mechanism, together with the vise, thus constituted a crude but efficient universal joint for holding the specimens in any desired position.

The specimen was placed in the apparatus; the calcaneus was clamped first, with the presumed plane of the axis of rotation perpendicular to the floor. The point of rotation on the talus was first located roughly by the unaided eye, then the binocular microscope was swung into position, and the talar axis point was accurately determined. The specimen was reversed 180°, with the talus clamped in the apparatus and the above procedure repeated to determine the calcaneal terminus of the axis. A check on the accuracy of axis location by this method was accomplished by attaching a red filter to the binocular microscope and marking the axis points with a red pencil. Four separate runs were made on each of five random specimens; all five points were run once on four successive days (to prevent memorization of bone contours). All markings on all five specimens were found to coincide within 3 mm. After the rotation points were found, brass escutcheon pins (16 mm long) were driven up to the head into the individual bones, thus marking the points of emergence of the axis of the subtalar joint on the dorsum of the talus and the posterolateral surface of the calcaneus.

With the calcaneus supported with bits of cardboard, the bones were articulated and inclined so that the plane of the axis was horizontal to the eye. X-rays were secured of each of the pairs of the articulated bones. The distance of the x-ray tube from the specimen was 61 cm and was centered over the posterior facet of the calcaneus (Fig. I-3).

In such an orientation, the posterior facet is almost vertical as viewed in the lateral projection (Fig. I-3) and appears in the dorsiplantar projection as a relatively straight articular crevice (Fig. I-4).

If the anatomic arrangement of the posterior articular facet is such as to generate a screwlike movement between the talus and the calcaneus (as one bone is rotated upon the other), then the plane of the posterior facet as viewed in the dorsiplantar projection (Fig. I-5) should form an angle (helix angle, α) with the plane at the axis of rotation. The "helix angle of a thread" of a screw is defined as the angle made

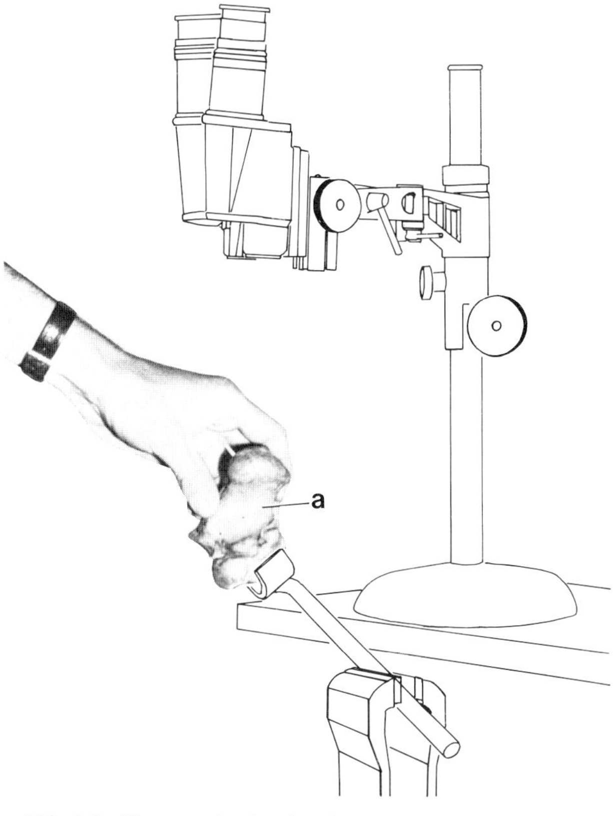

FIG. I-2. Photograph showing bones reversed. *a*, Calcaneus rotated on fixed talus. The point of minimal motion is located and marked on the calcaneus.

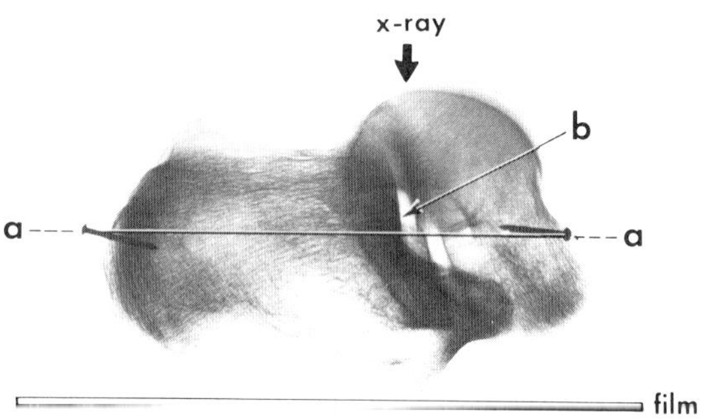

FIG. I-3. Lateral roentgenogram of articulated talus and calcaneus (dried bones). *Line a——a* connects two escutcheon pins representing empirically located axis. *b*, Interval depicting posterior articulation between talus and calcaneus. It should be noted that this interval lies in a plane that is almost perpendicular to the plane of the axis. The direction of the beam of the x-ray used in Figure I-4 is represented by the *arrow;* the film is located below the specimen.

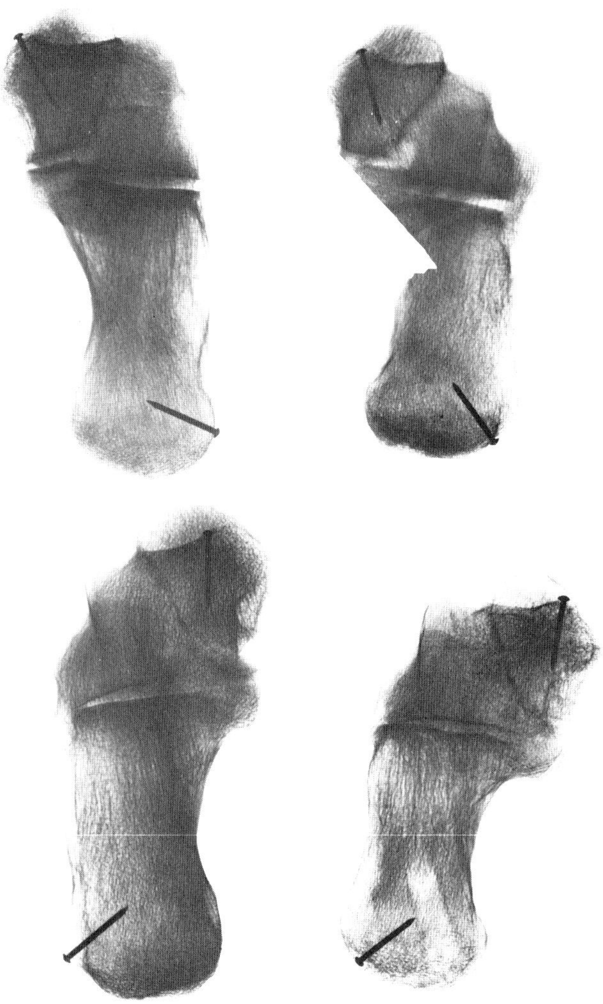

FIG. I-4. X-rays of four randomly selected articulated tali and calcanei, in projection depicted in Figure I-3. Note that the posterior facet of the talocalcaneal articulation appears as a relatively straight crevice.

between the helix (spiral) of the thread at the pitch diameter and a line perpendicular to the axis. The pitch diameter is defined as the diameter of an imaginary cylinder lying midway between the major (outside) diameter and the minor (root) diameter. In the roentgenograms it is impossible to determine the pitch diameter and thus determine the precise helix angle. However, it was felt that the inclination of the posterior facet (as depicted in the roentgenograms) to the empirically located subtalar axis could be utilized to approximate the helix angle roughly, particularly since absolute values were not being sought, but only the amounts of individual variations that would be encountered in a small randomly selected sample.

The angle between the posterior facet and a line perpendicular to the empirically located axis of the subtalar joint was found to be 24.7° ± 7.6°, with a range of 2 to 40°. If it is assumed that this angle as measured approximates the helix angle, the average value in our series is twice that reported by Manter. However, this angle shows considerable variation between individual specimens, and Manter's "average" for a small sample could fall well within the ranges found in our series of 50 specimens.

An observation on the relationship of the posterior facet to the trabecular pattern of the calcaneus was inadvertently noted when the x-rays of the 50 isolated tali and calcanei were reviewed (see above). The trabeculae of the calcaneus appeared to be essentially parallel and perpendicular to the joint margin of the posterior facet (Fig. I-4). To substantiate this casual observation the angle between a line drawn on the x-rays paralleling the trabeculae and a line representing the joint surface was measured in the 50 x-rays.

This angle was found to be surprisingly constant. It measured 92° ± 5° with a maximal deviation of only 9° from the average (Fig. I-6). This is remarkable since the accuracy of the lines drawn on the x-rays was always a matter of personal judgment. Unfortunately lateral x-rays were obtained in only six of the 50 specimens, but in these the trabecular pattern also appeared to approach the articular surface at a right angle (Fig. I-3).

If it is assumed that the trabeculae represent the direction of the major forces transmitted through the calcaneus, then it is interesting to find that the posterior facet is so positioned that it receives these forces as compression forces directed at right angles to the articular surface and that they therefore can not seriously affect free movement of the joint while it is under load. Furthermore, it appears reasonable to conclude from these findings that during growth the final orientation of the posterior facet of the subtalar joint is dependent more upon the forces transmitted through the joint than upon its axis of movement.

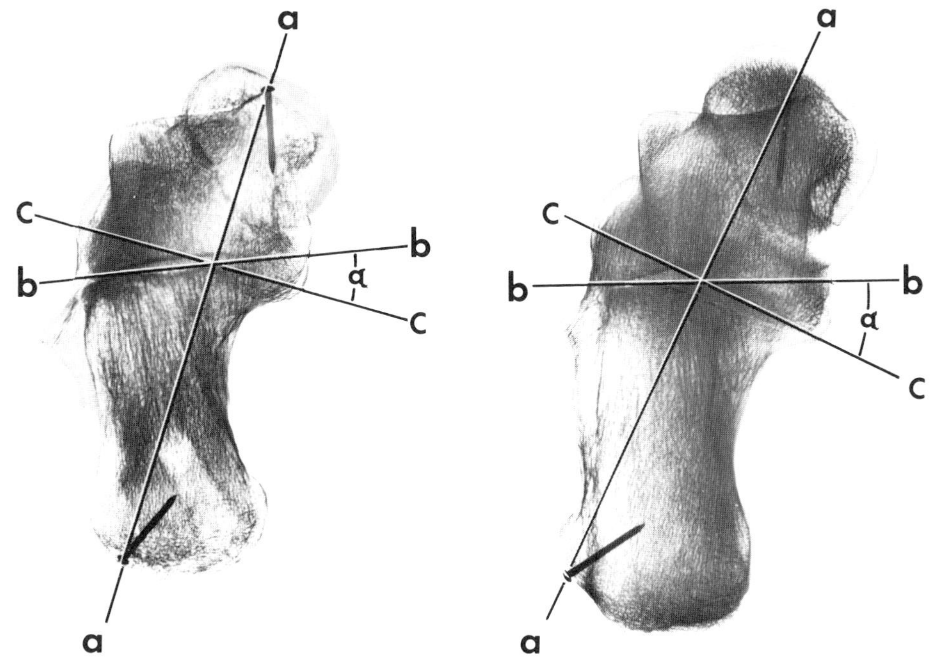

FIG. I-5. Method of estimating helix angle. *Line a——a* connects heads of escrutcheon pins, denoting axis of subtalar joint. *Line b——b* is drawn parallel to sides of crevice representing posterior facet of talocalcaneal articulation. *Line c——c* is drawn perpendicular to *line a——a*. α, assumed helix angle, which is measured.

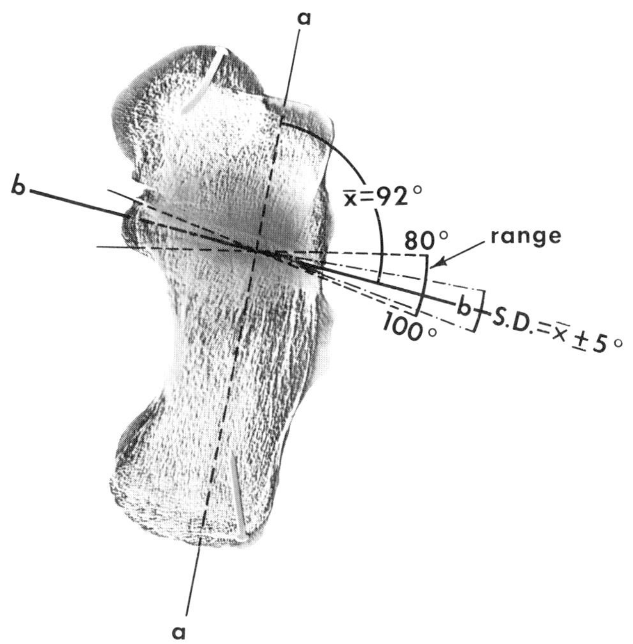

FIG. I-6. Bas relief showing relation of trabeculae of calcaneus to posterior facet of subtalar joint. *Line a——a* is parallel to trabeculae of calcaneus. *Line b——b* is drawn parallel to crevice representing posterior facet of talocalcaneal articulation. The angle between the two lines was measured and was found to approximate 90°.

appendix J

ranges of motion at the subtalar joint

This Appendix describes the techniques employed in the study on the ranges of motion in the subtalar joint. The studies were carried out on cadaver material and on living individuals.

Cadaver Studies

This section reports on two independent studies done three years apart by different investigators, on two separate series of cadaver feet. The first series consisted of 47 and the second of 102 specimens. They are reported separately.

Series I (47 specimens). The calcaneus and talus were removed together from cadaver feet. All soft tissues were removed except the capsular and ligamentous structures connecting the two bones. The axis of the subtalar joint was located and a stainless steel pin inserted in the usual manner (Appendix F). The calcaneus was held in a vise and the talus remained free to rotate about the empirically located axis. A protractor was mounted on and perpendicular to the stainless steel axis that protruded from the talus. A 0.5 mm stainless steel pin was drilled into the head of the talus, parallel to the plane of the protractor. The talus was rotated through its full range of possible motion and the angle of this total motion was recorded. The embalming process obviously resulted in some restriction of motion, particularly as a result of loss of elasticity in the interosseous talocalcaneal ligament. Therefore, all ligaments were carefully removed and the ranges of motion again recorded with the talus free to move on the calcaneus without the restriction of any ligamentous structures. The joint was rotated through its full range with manual pressure to keep the articulating surfaces in contact, extremes of movement being limited by osseous contact. Obviously the first series of measurements was probably less than normal while the second series may have demonstrated excessive motion.

The average amount of motion in the first series of measurements was 18° ± 6°, with a range of 10 to 41°. In the second series of measurements the average was 36° ± 10°, with a range of 17 to 59°.

Series II (102 specimens). The cadaver specimens utilized in the investigation of the screwlike movement between the talus and calcaneus (Appendix F) also yielded data on the range of motion at the subtalar joint. The extremes of motion were terminated when articular cartilage of the talus no longer contacted the articular surface of the posterior facet of the calcaneus.

In this series the right and left sides were recorded separately to determine whether any obvious differences would appear, but none were seen. The results are shown in Table J-1.

Table J-1. Range of motion at subtalar joint

Subtalar joint	No. of specimens	Average	Range
Right	48	24.7° ± 10.6°	5 to 54°
Left	54	23.2 ± 11.4	4 to 55
Total	102	24 ± 11	4 to 55

Normal Subjects

The total range of motion in the subtalar joint was determined in an unselected group of 50 subjects. Both right and left feet were measured, providing data on 100 feet. There were 14 men and 36 women. The age range was 22 to 62 years, with an average of 34 years. None of the subjects gave a history of fractures or sprains about the ankle or of persistent foot pain, nor were any deformities revealed on examination or any abnormalities of gait demonstrated.

The technique for measuring the range of motion was based upon the positioning of the foot and the use of a specially constructed spherical goniometer. Both the positioning of the foot and the construction and use of the goniometer require more detailed discussion.

Ideally, the motion between the talus and the calcaneus should be measured in a plane that is at a right angle to the axis of rotation. However, the position of the axis has been shown to be variable and in the living can only be roughly estimated. An attempt was made to achieve measurements that were as accurate as possible by employing a specially constructed spherical goniometer and utilizing "set" positions of the leg and foot.

Spherical Goniometer. A glass sphere, 5 cm in diameter, was the basic element of the goniometer. It was filled with water and sealed, except for a tiny air bubble with a diameter of approximately 2 mm (Fig. J-1). This provided a type of level in which the bubble remained always in a vertical position over the center of the sphere, no matter how the sphere was tilted or

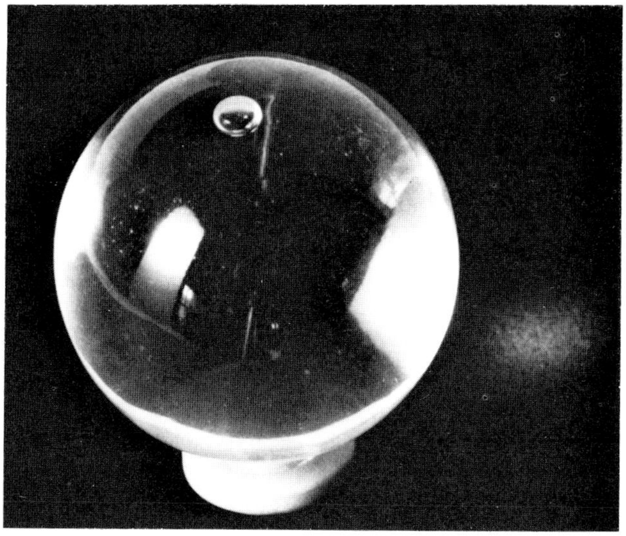

FIG. J-1. Basic element of spherical goniometer. A glass sphere is filled with water and sealed. A small bubble of air remains that can move along any great circle pathway within the sphere and always remain vertical to the center of the sphere, no matter what rotational displacement occurs.

rotated. A movable scale was fitted over the sphere and glued to two sectors of a sphere of clear plastic. This arrangement permitted the scale to be moved while always lying in a meridian of the spherical level. When used, the spherical goniometer was fixed to a laminated plastic heel cup (Fig. J-2*A*) or a molded plastic platform for application to the dorsum of the foot (Fig. J-2*B*). The methods of application of the goniometers to the foot are shown in Figure J-3, *A* and *B*.

Positioning of the Foot. To assure that the measurements obtained from the spherical goniometer would be reasonably accurate, the axis of the subtalar joint should be as nearly horizontal as possible. To achieve this, two positions of the leg and foot were utilized. The subject first was placed prone and the knee flexed to 135°, the foot being kept at a right angle to the lower leg. Since the average inclination of the axis is around 45°, this position places the axis approximately in a horizontal plane. Knee flexion relaxed the gastrocnemius and obviated any restrictive influence that it might exert on the free movement of the subtalar joint. The second position consisted of having the subject sit on the edge of the examining table with the knee flexed to 90°. The foot was passively plantar flexed to approximately 45°. This maneuver again places the average subtalar axis in approximately a horizontal plane (Fig. J-4).

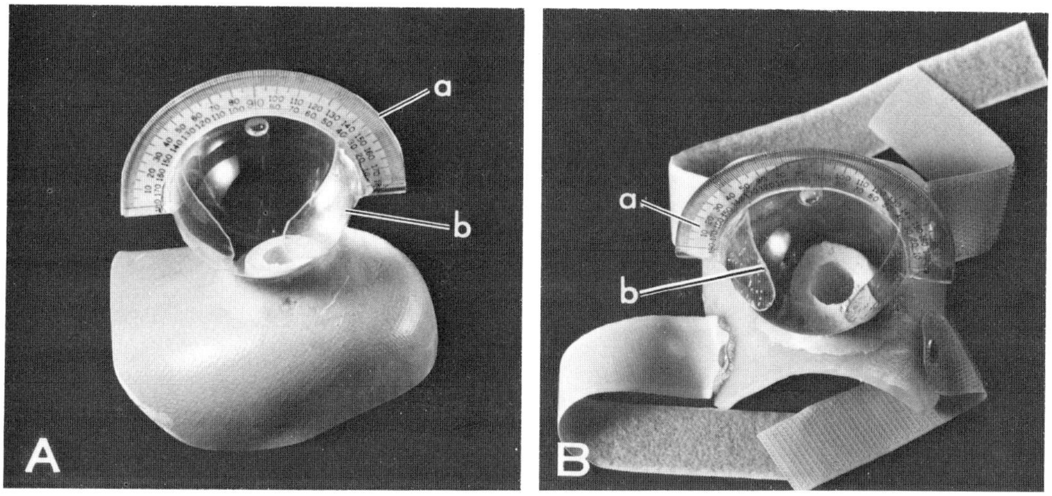

FIG. J-2. Completely assembled spherical goniometers for determination of ranges of motion in subtalar joints. *a*, Scales glued to two sectors of sphere (*b*). These scales can be moved to overlie any pathway of travel of the bubble. *A*, Spherical goniometer glued to laminated heel cup. *B*, Spherical goniometer glued to molded laminated platform for application to dorsum of foot. Straps of Velcro have been provided for firm fixation of the platform to the foot.

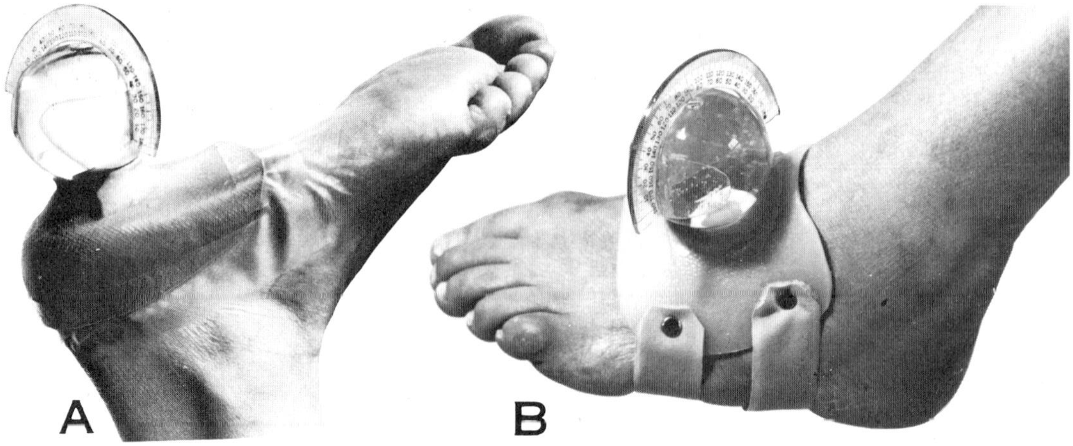

FIG. J-3. Attachment of goniometers to foot. *A*, Laminated heel cup firmly taped to skin of heel. *B*, Laminated plastic platform held rigidly in place on dorsum of foot by means of two straps of Velcro.

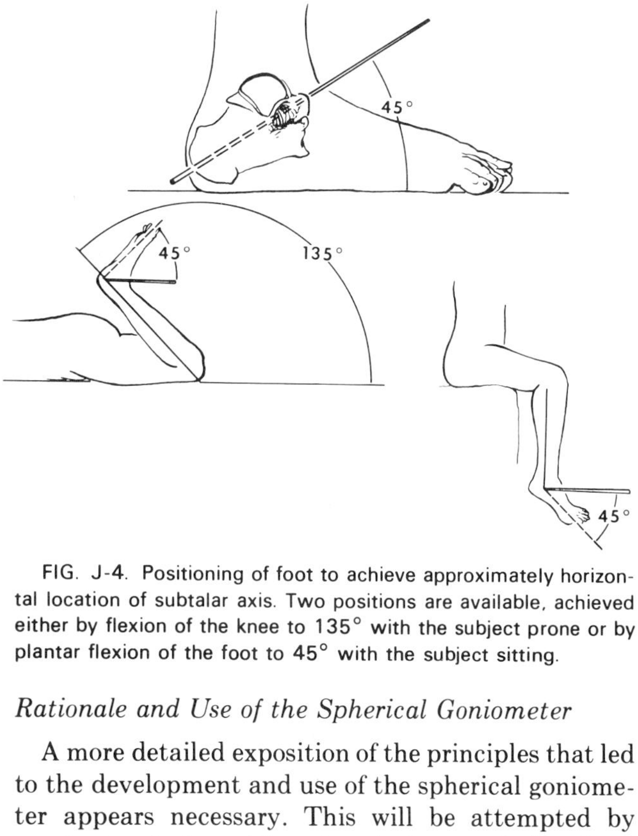

FIG. J-4. Positioning of foot to achieve approximately horizontal location of subtalar axis. Two positions are available, achieved either by flexion of the knee to 135° with the subject prone or by plantar flexion of the foot to 45° with the subject sitting.

Rationale and Use of the Spherical Goniometer

A more detailed exposition of the principles that led to the development and use of the spherical goniometer appears necessary. This will be attempted by employing both written descriptions and drawings. The presentation will be sequential, starting with basic concepts and progressing to the practical application of the device.

The use of gravity to establish one arm of the angle to be measured accomplished two purposes. It obviated the need to locate precisely the axis of rotation, and the goniometer could be located at any distance from the axis. This is demonstrated in the sketch with the use of plumb bobs (Fig. J-5). A spherical level acts in the same manner as does a plumb bob.

The accuracy of the measurement of the rotation obviously depends upon the axis remaining in a horizontal plane. This is attempted by placing the subject in first one and then the other of the two positions (see Fig. J-4). Unfortunately it can not be determined whether in any individual the positioning of the foot in space assures that the axis is precisely horizontal. The anthropometric studies indicate that the axis may vary 20° on either side of the mean of 42°. In both situations the angle measured will be less than the actual amount of rotation. This decrease in the measured angle will vary as the cosine of the angle of deviation of the axis from the horizontal. Reference to trigonometric tables indicates that the maximal error involved is probably less than 10%.

It should be noted that the axis of the subtalar joint also varies in the transverse plane, being inclined medially from the midline of the foot from 4 to 48°. The spherical goniometer automatically accommodates this variation with rotation. The bubble will move through an arc of a great circle that is perpendicular to the axis of motion. All that is necessary is to adjust the movable scale over the sphere so that it lies in the plane of travel of the bubble. The procedure employed in measuring the range of motion in the subtalar joint with the spherical goniometer was as follows.

1. The subject was placed prone with the knee flexed to 135° and the foot held at a right angle to the leg.

2. A snugly fitting heel cup carrying the spherical goniometer was taped securely to the heel of the subject.

3. The forefoot was maximally inverted and everted passively by the examiner. The rotatory forces were applied to the forefoot in such a way as not to cause any displacement of the heel cup on the heel.

The path of the bubble was noted and the scale was moved so as to lie over the path of travel of the bubble. The total angular movement was noted and recorded (Fig. J-6).

4. The subject was next asked to sit on the edge of the table with the knee flexed to 90° and the foot plantar flexed approximately 45°. A second goniometer was taped to the dorsum of the foot.

5. By grasping the heel, the examiner forcibly inverted and everted the heel. The remainder of the foot followed the displacement of the heel passively (Fig. J-7).

6. The movement of the bubble was again noted and the scale was adjusted to overlie the path of the bubble.

7. The angular displacement with passive maximal inversion and eversion of the heel was noted and recorded.

Differences in measurements as recorded from heel and forefoot occurred in most subjects, but they rarely exceeded 10°. The range of motion measured with the goniometer on the heel tended to be greater than the motion recorded with the goniometer on the dorsum of the foot. Histograms of the measurements revealed nearly perfect distribution curves.

The average range of motion with the goniometer on the heel was 44° ± 7°, with a range of 24 to 65°. The average range of motion with the goniometer on the

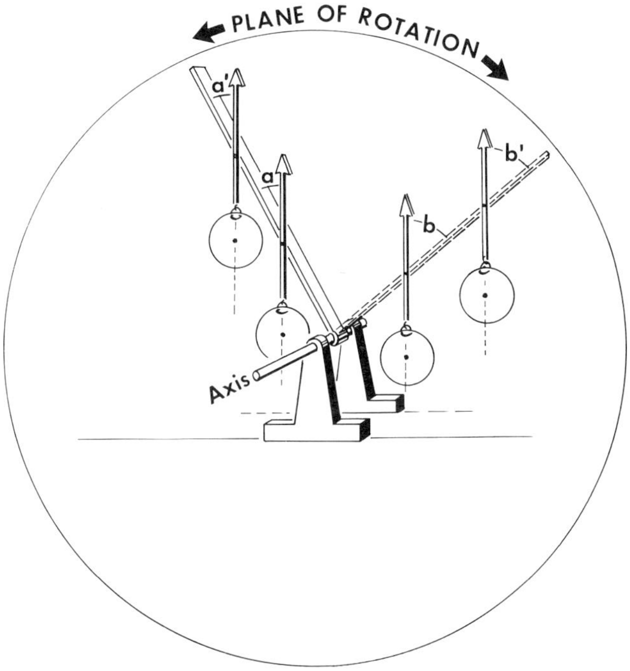

FIG. J-5. Diagrammatic demonstration of principle underlying use of spherical goniometer. Plumb bobs have been mounted at varying distances on arms extending from a horizontal axis. Since the axis is horizontal and the plumb bobs are always vertical the angles will remain equal no matter how far removed from the axis of rotation ($<a = <a'$ and $<b = <b'$). The *circle* at the bottom of each pendulum represents the spherical goniometer. The sphere is filled with fluid except for a small bubble which will always align itself vertically with the center of the sphere, and thus behave in a manner similar to that of a plumb bob. Obviously, because of its spherical construction the bubble is free to move in several planes, making it more versatile than a plumb bob, which records accurately in only one plane. After application of the spherical goniometer to the foot, the pathway of the bubble along an arc of a great circle is noted and a movable scale is aligned to the path of travel.

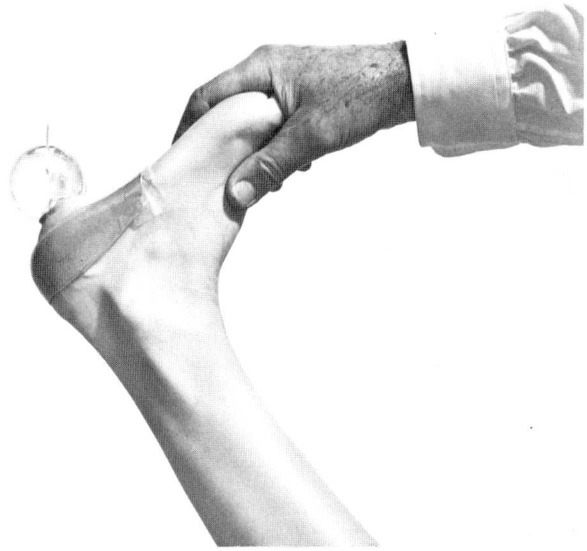

FIG. J-6. Spherical goniometer in use. The heel cup carrying the goniometer has been taped securely to the heel. With the leg stabilized by one hand of the examiner the other hand inverts and everts the forefoot while maintaining the foot at a right angle to the leg. The excursion of the bubble is measured on the circular scale.

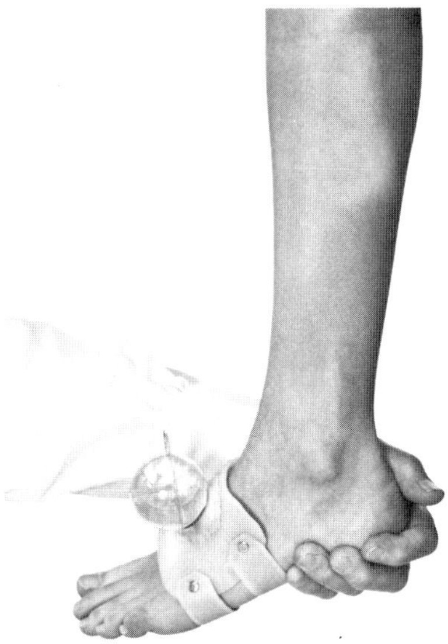

FIG. J-7. Motion in subtalar joint being checked by measuring motion of forefoot. The spherical goniometer has been strapped to the foot. The examiner rotates the heel, and the excursion of the bubble is measured on the circular scale.

dorsum of the foot was 36° ± 8°, with a range of 20 to 50°. If the two measurements are combined the average range of motion is approximately 40°, with a range of 20 to 62°. Scatter diagrams indicated no correlation between ranges of motion and sex or age in this series.

Attention is directed to the differences in the values for the average amount of motion in the subtalar joint obtained from the cadaver studies as compared with those in the living. The cadaver studies yielded averages which are approximately half as large as those calculated from measurements on the living. Several explanations for these differences are possible. A review of the data from each of the studies reveals that the maximal amounts of motion recorded in all three studies were comparable (55, 59, and 65°). However, in the cadaver studies the minimal amount of movement was far less than in the living. Recorded measurements of only a few degrees of motion were frequent in the cadaver specimens, while the minimal amount of motion recorded in the living was 20°. The presence of smaller measurements would naturally tend to lower the average value of the range of motion in the cadaver series. These smaller measurements on the amount of motion in the cadaver might have resulted from embalming, but conversely, the motion measured on the living might have been excessive. Several factors might be mentioned that could contribute to abnormally large measurements as recorded in the living. The joints were passively moved by the investigator and the articular surfaces were not under compression, thus possibly permitting abnormal separation of the joint surfaces at the extremes of movement. The goniometer could not be fixed rigidly to the bony structures, and the displacement of the goniometer was necessarily carried out through soft tissues. Therefore, movement in joints other than the subtalar joint may have occurred. Assuming that the true value for the average range of motion in the subtalar joint lies somewhere between 24 and 44°, this amount of motion is two to three times that commonly quoted in the literature.

appendix K

relation of the calcaneal tendon to the subtalar axis

Most careful investigators agree that the most mobile joints in the foot (ignoring the toes) are the three articulations of the hindfoot (together, the talocalcaneocuboid joint). These articulations constitute a closed kinematic chain (Huson, 1973) and there exists an interdependence of movement between them. Fixation of one joint blocks the mobility of the other two joints, and movement of one of the joints compels the others to move. Of the three articulations, the subtalar (talocalcaneal) is the most mobile and the most important (Inkster, 1938; Shephard, 1951). During the latter part of stance phase when the heel is rising in preparation for push-off, the principal muscle acting upon the subtalar joint is the triceps surae. Its ability to produce an inverting moment depends upon its effective lever arm (which is the distance between the axis of the subtalar joint and the insertion of the calcaneal tendon). To determine the length of the effective lever arm and its variations within the population, the following measurements were carried out on cadaver feet.

One hundred two calcanei were available for study. The axes of their subtalar joints had previously been determined (see Appendix F). To measure the distances between the axis and the calcaneal tendon it was necessary to clean the tendon of extraneous tissue so as to reveal clearly its insertion and to modify a sliding caliper to obtain the required measurements. A commercially available caliper was modified in the following manner (Fig. K-1). To the fixed jaw of the caliper a 3-mm stainless steel rod was attached. This rod was for insertion into the drill hole in the calcaneus which had been previously made where the axis of the subtalar joint had been empirically determined. The placement of the rod assured that the distance measured was perpendicular to the axis of the joint. Three stainless steel extensions were added to the movable jaw of the caliper. These were necessary since the axis of the subtalar joint often emerged some distance from the tendon and the regular jaw of the caliper was too short to reach the edges of the tendon. Furthermore, lining up the extensions by eye in a plane paralleling the calcaneal tendon assured that the distances measured closely approached the true lengths of the effective lever arms. The following steps were taken to obtain the measurements of the effective lever arms.

1. The sliding calipers were modified as shown in Figure K-1.

2. The calcanei were cleaned of excessive soft tissue to reveal the insertion of the calcaneal tendon clearly.

3. The 3-mm stainless steel rod attached to the fixed jaw of the caliper was inserted into the drill hole previously made which located the empirically determined axis of the subtalar joint (Appendix F).

4. The caliper was rotated so that the three extensions on the movable jaw lay in a plane paralleling the calcaneal tendon (Fig. K-2). Three measurements were taken: the three distances from the axis rod to the lateral edge of the tendon, to the medial edge of the tendon, and to the middle of the tendon. In addition, the width of the tendon at its insertion was measured by reversing the caliper and employing the inside jaws (Fig. K-3).

It was immediately apparent at the start of the measurements that in approximately half of the specimens, the lateral edge of the calcaneal tendon extended laterally beyond the axis of the subtalar joint. Therefore it was necessary to tabulate the measurements as positive values when the lateral edge lay medial to the axis and as negative values when the lateral edge of the tendon extended lateral to the axis.

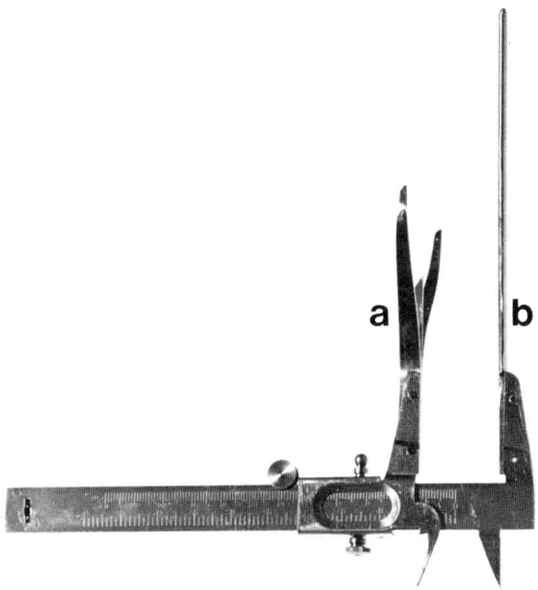

FIG. K-1. Modified, sliding caliper. *a*, Three extensions fixed to movable jaw, *b*, 3-mm stainless steel rod attached to fixed jaw of caliper.

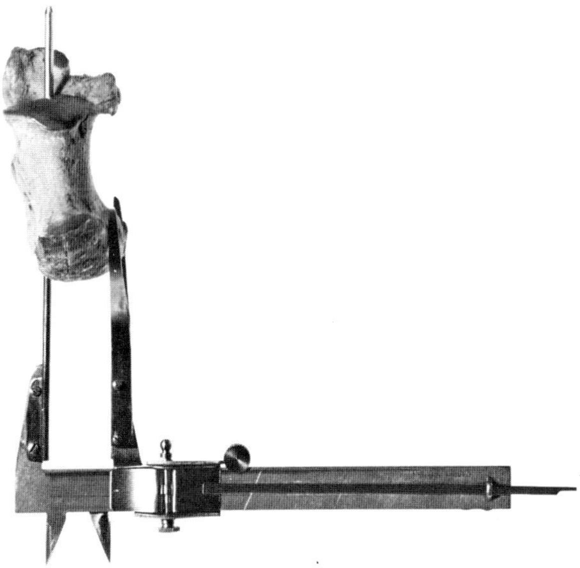

FIG. K-2. Modified caliper in use. The 3-mm rod has been inserted into the hole previously drilled to correspond to the empirically located axis of the subtalar joint (Appendix F). The extensions on the movable jaw are adjusted to lie in a plane paralleling the calcaneal tendon and contacting the medial edge of the tendon. The length of the effective lever is read to the nearest millimeter from the scale on the caliper.

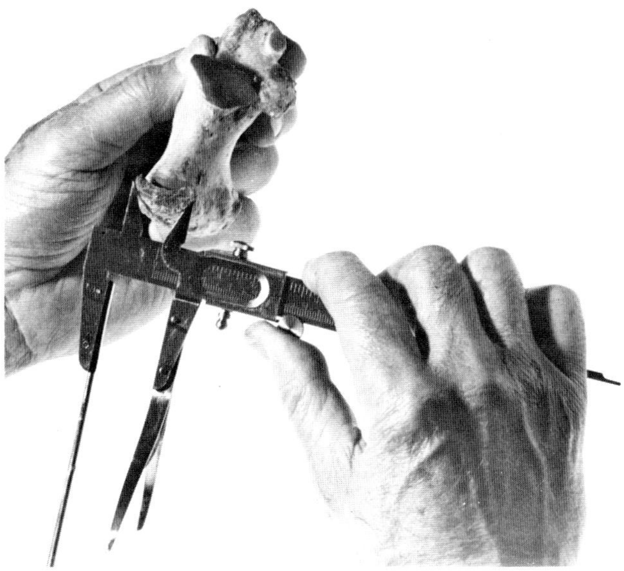

FIG. K-3. Measurement of width of calcaneal tendon. By reversing the caliper and using the inside jaws the anatomic width of the tendon was measured.

The average width of the calcaneal tendon at its insertion was ± 19.9 mm, with a range of 12 to 27 mm.

The average distance from the lateral edge of the calcaneal tendon to the axis of the subtalar joint was -0.15 mm ± 4.9 mm, with a range of 9 to -12 mm.

The average distance from the medial edge of the calcaneal tendon to the axis of the subtalar joint was 19.7 mm ± 5.4 mm, with a range of 37 to 10 mm.

The average distance from the center of the calcaneal tendon to the axis of the subtalar joint was 10 mm ± 2 mm.

A review of the data indicates that in half of the specimens the axis of the subtalar joint passed within 2 mm of the lateral edge of the calcaneal tendon at its insertion. In the remainder, the axis passed more than 2 mm medial or lateral to the lateral edge of the calcaneal tendon.

Because of the width of the calcaneal tendon, the place may be chosen arbitrarily which may be assumed to be the point of concentration of the force and hence provide a spot for measurement of the effective lever arm. A reasonable assumption appears to be the middle of the tendon. In this case an effective lever arm of approximately 1 cm, on the average, may be postulated. Therefore tension transmitted to the calcaneus will produce an inversion moment on the heel. However, the variations in this assumed lever arm are considerable. In some specimens the inversion moment may be minimal as a result of a negligible lever arm (less than 2 mm), while in other specimens the inversion moment must be large since the lever arm is long (the maximal recorded length was 21 mm).

references

Alezais. La torsion du tendon d'Achille chez l'homme. *C. R. Soc. Biol. (Paris) 51:* 728, 1899.

Alldredge, R. H. Diastasis of the distal tibiofibular joint and associated lesions. *J.A.M.A. 115:* 2136, 1940.

Allen, H. *A System of Human Anatomy, Including its Medical and Surgical Relations.* Henry C. Lea's Son & Company, Philadelphia, 1882.

Anderson, K. J., and LeCocq, J. F. Operative treatment of injury to the fibular collateral ligament of the ankle. *J. Bone Joint Surg. 36-A:* 825, 1954.

Ashhurst, A. P. C., and Bromer, R. S. Classification and mechanism of fractures of the leg bones involving the ankle, based on a study of three hundred cases from the Episcopal Hospital: Anatomic and surgical study. *Arch. Surg. 4:* 51, 1922.

Attenborough, C. G. Severe congenital talipes equinovarus. *J. Bone Joint Surg. 48-B:* 31, 1966.

Bairati, A. *Trattato di anatomia umana: Morfologia generale e sistematica dell'uomo,* vol. 4. Minerva Medica, Turin, 1963.

Barnett, C. H., and Napier, J. R. The axis of rotation at the ankle joint in man: Its influence upon the form of the talus and the mobility of the fibula. *J. Anat. 86:* 1, 1952.

Benninghoff-Goerttler. *Lehrbuch der Anatomie des Menschen, dargestellt unter Bevorzugung funktioneller Zusammenhänge,* edited by A. Benninghoff and K. Goerttler, ed. 7, vol. 1. Urban & Schwarzenberg, Munich, Berlin, 1960.

Bergmann, G. A. Die Bedeutung der Innendrehung der Unterschenkel für die Entwicklung des Senk-Knickfusses mit der Angabe einer Messmethode der Unterschenkeltorsion und Mitteilung von Messergebnissen. *Z. Orthop. 96:* 177, 1962.

Berndt, A. L., and Harty, M. Transchondral fractures (osteochondritis dissecans) of the talus. *J. Bone Joint Surg. 41-A:* 988, 1959.

Berry, F. R., Jr. *Angle Variation Patterns of Normal Hip, Knee and Ankle in Different Operations.* Prosthetic Devices Research Project, Institute of Engineering Research, University of California, Berkeley. Series 11, issue 21. The Project, Berkeley, 1952.

Bíró, B., and Tarsoly, E. Über die Struktur der Achillessehne. *Beitr. Orthop. Traumatol. 14:* 682, 1967.

Bland-Sutton, J. *Ligaments: Their Nature and Morphology,* ed. 2. H. K. Lewis, London, 1897.

Bonnin, J. G. Editorials and annotations: Injury to the ligaments of the ankle. *J. Bone Joint Surg. 47-B:* 609, 1965.

Braune, W., and Fischer, O. Die Bewegungen des Kniegelenks, nach einer neuen Methode am lebenden Menschen gemessen. *Abh. math.-phys. Classe K. Sächs. Ges. Wissensch. 17:* 75, 1891.

Braus, H. *Anatomie des Menschen: Ein Lehrbuch für Studierende und Ärzte,* ed. 3, vol. 1. Springer-Verlag, Berlin, 1954.

Bromfeild, W. *Chirurgical Observations and Cases,* vol. 2. T. Cadell, London, 1773.

Buchholz, H.-W. Personal communication, 1974.

Burrows. H. J. Fatigue fractures of the fibula. *J. Bone Joint Surg. 30-B:* 266, 1948.

Cailliet, R. *Foot and Ankle Pain.* F. A. Davis Company, Philadelphia, 1968.

Charpy, A., Nicolas, A., Prenant, A., Poirier, P., Jacques, P., and Rieffel. *Traité d'anatomie humaine,* edited by P. Poirier and A. Charpy, ed. 2, vol. 1. Masson & Cie, Paris, 1899.

Clark, A. E. *The Ankle Joint of Man.* M. D. Thesis, University of Berne, Berne, 1877.

Clark, M. E. Morphology of the Achilles tendon in the newborn. *J. Am. Podiatry Assoc. 62:* 389, 1972.

Close, J. R. Some applications of the functional anatomy of the ankle joint. *J. Bone Joint Surg. 38-A:* 761, 1956.

Close, J. R., and Inman, V. T. *The Action of the Ankle Joint.* Prosthetic Devices Research Project, Institute of Engineering Research, University of California, Berkeley. Series 11, issue 22. The Project, Berkeley, 1952.

Colonna, P. C. *Regional Orthopedic Surgery.* W. B. Saunders Company, Philadelphia, 1950.

Costigan, P. G. Treatment of true widening of ankle mortise. *Can. Med. Assoc. J. 69:* 310, 1953.

Cummins, E. J., Anson, B. J., Carr, B. W., and Wright, R. R. The structure of the calcaneal tendon (of Achilles) in relation to orthopedic surgery, with additional observations on the plantaris muscle. *Surg. Gynecol. Obstet. 83:* 107, 1946.

Cunningham, D. J. *Text-Book of Anatomy,* ed. 2. William Wood and Company, New York, 1905.

Cunningham, D. J. *Cunningham's Text-Book of Anatomy,* edited by Arthur Robinson, ed. 5. William Wood and Company, New York, 1927.

Cunningham, D. J. *Cunningham's Textbook of Anatomy,* edited by G. J. Romanes, ed. 10. Oxford University Press, London, 1964.

D'Aubigné, R. M., and Smets, W. Les formes frustes de déplacement externe de l'astragale. *Presse méd. 42:* 157, 1934.

Devas, M. B., and Sweetnam, R. Stress fractures of the fibula: A review of fifty cases in athletes. *J. Bone Joint Surg. 38-B:* 818, 1956.

Dönitz, A. *Die Mechanik der Fusswurzel.* M. D. Thesis, Friedrich-Wilhelms-Universität, Berlin, 1903.

Dunn, H. K., and Samuelson, K. M. Flat-top talus: A long-term report of twenty club feet. *J. Bone Joint Surg. 56-A:* 57, 1974.

(DuVries, H. L.) *DuVries' Surgery of the Foot,* edited by V. T. Inman, ed. 3. The C. V. Mosby Company, St. Louis, 1973.

Elftman, H., and Manter, J. The evolution of the human foot, with especial reference to the joints. *J. Anat. 70:* 56, 1935.

Elmslie, R. C. Recurrent subluxation of the ankle-joint. *Ann. Surg. 100:* 364, 1934.

Fick, R. *Handbuch der Anatomie und Mechanik der Gelenke unter Berücksichtigung der bewegenden Muskeln,* Part 1. Gustav Fischer Verlag, Jena, 1904.

Francillon, M. R. Distorsio pedis with an isolated lesion of the ligamentum calcaneo-fibulare. *Acta Orthop. Scand. 32:* 469, 1962.

Frazer, J. E. The Anatomy of the Human Skeleton. J. & A. Churchill, London, 1933.

Frazer's Anatomy of the Human Skeleton. J. & A. Churchill, London, 1965.

Gardner, E., Gray, D. J., and O'Rahilly, R. *Anatomy: A Regional Study of Human Structure*, ed. 3. W. B. Saunders Company, Philadelphia, 1969.

Golebiewski. Studien über die Ausdehnungsfähigkeit des menschlichen Fusses. *Z. Orthop. Chir. 3:* 243, 1894.

Gordon, R. B. Arthrography of the ankle joint: Experience in one hundred seven studies. *J. Bone Joint Surg. 52-A:* 1623, 1970.

Grant, J. C. B. *Grant's Method of Anatomy: By Regions, Descriptive and Deductive*, edited by J. V. Basmajian, ed. 8. The Williams & Wilkins Company, Baltimore, 1971.

Grath, G.-B. Widening of the ankle mortise: A clinical and experimental study. *Acta Chir. Scand. (suppl. 263)* 1960.

Gray, H. *Anatomy: Descriptive and Surgical.* John W. Parker & Son, London, 1858.

Gray, H. *Anatomy of the Human Body*, edited by C. M. Goss, ed. 29. Lea & Febiger, Philadelphia, 1973.

Griffiths, A. L. Fatigue fracture of the fibula in childhood. *Arch. Dis. Child. 27:* 552, 1952.

Gustilo, R. B., and Gordon, S. S. Osteochondral fractures of the talus (osteochondritis dissecans). *Minn. Med. 51:* 237, 1968.

Henke, J. W. Die Bewegung des Fusses am Sprungbein. *Z. rationelle Med. (n.s.) 7:* 225, 1855.

Henke, J. W. *Handbuch der Anatomie und Mechanik der Gelenke.* C. F. Winter'sche Verlagshandlung, Leipzig, 1863.

Henle, J. *Handbuch der systematischen Anatomie des Menschen*, ed. 3, vol. 1. Friedrich Vieweg, Braunschweig, 1871.

Hicks, J. H. The mechanics of the foot. I. The joints. *J. Anat. 87:* 345, 1953.

Hicks, J. H. The mechanics of the foot. II. The plantar aponeurosis and the arch. *J. Anat. 88:* 25, 1954.

Hill, W. C. O. *Primates: Comparative Anatomy and Taxonomy*, vol. 4, part A. Edinburgh University Press, Edinburgh, 1960.

Hollinshead, W. H. *Textbook of Anatomy*, ed. 2. Harper and Row, New York, 1967.

Horner, W. E. *A Treatise on Special and General Anatomy*, ed. 4. Carey, Lea & Blanchard, Philadelphia, 1836.

Howorth, M. B. *A Textbook of Orthopedics, with a Section on Neurology in Orthopedics.* W. B. Saunders Company, Philadelphia, 1952.

Hsu, L. C. S., Yau, A. C. M. C., O'Brien, J. P., and Hodgson, A. R. Valgus deformity of the ankle resulting from fibular resection for a graft in subtalar fusion in children. *J. Bone Joint Surg. 54-A:* 585, 1972.

Humphry, G. M. *A Treatise on the Human Skeleton (Including the Joints).* Macmillan and Co., Cambridge, 1858.

Huson, A. *Een ontleedkundig-functioneel onderzoek van de voetwortel: An Anatomical and Functional Study of the Tarsal Joints.* Luctor et Emergo, Leiden, 1961.

Huson, A. La chaîne cinématique fermée (importance de cette conception pour la mécanique articulaire). *C. R. Assoc. Anat. 57:* 887, 1973.

Hutter, C. G., Jr., and Scott, W. Tibial torsion. *J. Bone Joint Surg. 31-A:* 511, 1949.

Hyrtl, J. *Lehrbuch der Anatomie des Menschen, mit Rücksicht auf physiologische Begründung und praktische Anwendung*, ed. 12. Wilhelm Braumüller, Vienna, 1873.

Inkster, R. G. Inversion and eversion of the foot and the transverse tarsal joint. In Proceedings of the Anatomical Society of Great Britain and Ireland, May and June 1938. *J. Anat. 72:* 612, 1938.

Isman, R. E., and Inman, V. T. *Anthropometric Studies of the Human Foot and Ankle.* Biomechanics Laboratory, University of California, San Francisco and Berkeley. Technical Report 58. The Laboratory, San Francisco, 1968.

Jones, F. W. *Man's Place Among the Mammals.* Longmans, Green & Company, New York, 1929.

Jones, F. W. *Structure and Function as Seen in the Foot.* The Williams & Wilkins Company, Baltimore, 1944.

Junge, H., and von Känel, O. Typische Sprunggelenksveränderungen bei Fussballspielern. *Med. Welt 48:* 2576, 1964.

Keith, A. The ligaments of the catarrhine monkeys, with references to corresponding structures in man. *J. Anat. Physiol. 28 (n.s.8):* 149, 1893–1894.

Kelly, R. P. Ankle injuries. *Kentucky Med. J. 50:* 281, 1952.

Krause, W., Ed. *Handbuch der Anatomie des Menschen, mit einem Synonymenregister, auf Grundlage der neuen Baseler anatomischen Nomenclatur, unter Mitwirkung von W. His und W. Waldeyer und unter Verweisung auf den Handatlas der Anatomie von Werner Spalteholz.* Verlag von S. Hirzel, Leipzig, 1903.

Lambert, K. L. The weight-bearing function of the fibula: A strain gauge study. *J. Bone Joint Surg. 53-A:* 507, 1971.

Lane, W. A. The movements of the ankle-joint. *J. Anat. Physiol. (Lond.) 22:* 408, 1887–1888.

Lanz, T. von, and Wachsmuth, W. *Praktische Anatomie: Ein Lehr- und Hilfsbuch der anatomischen Grundlagen ärztlichen Handelns*, vol. 1, part 4. Springer-Verlag, Berlin, 1938.

Le Damany, P. La torsion du tibia: normale, pathologique, expérimentale. *J. Anat. Physiol. (Paris) 45:* 598, 1909.

Lee, H. G., and Horan, T. B. Internal fixation in injuries of the ankle. *Surg. Gynecol. Obstet. 76:* 593, 1948.

Leonard, M. H. Injuries of the lateral ligaments of the ankle: A clinical and experimental study. *J. Bone Joint Surg. 31-A:* 373, 1949.

Levens, A. S., Inman, V. T., and Blosser, J. A. Transverse rotation of the segments of the lower extremity in locomotion. *J. Bone Joint Surg. 30-A:* 859, 1948.

Lewin, P. *The Foot and Ankle*, ed. 2. Lea & Febiger, Philadelphia, 1941.

Luschka, H. von. *Die Anatomie der Glieder des Menschen*, vol. 3, part 1. Verlag der Lauppschen Buchhandlung, Tübingen, 1865.

Macalister, A. *A Text-Book of Human Anatomy: Systematic and Topographical, Including the Embryology, Histology, and Morphology of Man.* P. Blakiston, Son & Co., Philadelphia, 1889.

Makin, M. Tibio-fibular relationship in paralysed limbs. *J. Bone Joint Surg. 47-B:* 500, 1965.

Manter, J. T. Movements of the subtalar and transverse tarsal joints. *Anat. Rec. 80:* 397, 1941.

McMaster, J. H., and Scranton, P. E., Jr. Tibiofibular synostosis: A cause of ankle disability. (Paper no. 111) Presented at the Forty-second Annual Meeting of the American Academy of Orthopaedic Surgeons, San Francisco, March 1–6, 1975.

Meekison, M. Ankle injuries. In *The American Academy of Orthopaedic Surgeons Presents Lectures on Reconstruction Surgery, Selected from the Instructional Courses of the Twelfth Annual Assembly, Chicago, January 23–24, 1944*, edited by J. E. M. Thomson. J. W. Edwards, Ann Arbor, 1944.

Mensor, M. C., and Melody, G. F. Osteochondritis dissecans of ankle joint: The use of tomography as a diagnostic aid. *J. Bone Joint Surg. 23:* 903, 1941.

Meyer, G. H. von. Chap. 1: Ursache und Mechanismus der Entstehung des erworbenen Plattfusses, nebst Hinweisung auf die Indikationen zur Behandlung desselben. In *Studien über den Mechanismus des Fusses in normalen und abnormen Verhältnissen. Part 1: Der Plattfuss.* Verlag von Gustav Fischer, Jena, 1883.

Meyer, H. Das aufrechte Gehen (Zweiter Beitrag zur Mechanik des menschlichen Knochengerüstes). *Arch Anat. Physiol. wissensch. Med.*, p. 365, 1853.

Middleton, R. W. D. Ankle valgus due to fibular growth abnormality. *J. Bone Joint Surg. 57-B:* 118, 1975.

(Morris') Human Anatomy: A Complete Systematic Treatise by Various Authors, Including a Special Section on Surgical and

Topographical Anatomy, edited by H. Morris and M. B. Lond. P. Blakiston, Son & Co., Philadelphia, 1893.

Morris' Human Anatomy: A Complete Systematic Treatise, edited by B. J. Anson, ed. 12. The Blakiston Division, McGraw-Hill Book Company, New York, 1966.

Morris, J. M., and Blickenstaff, L. D. *Fatigue Fractures: A Clinical Study*. Charles C Thomas, Publisher, Springfield, Ill., 1967.

Mullins, J. F. P., and Sallis, J. G. Recurrent sprain of the ankle joint with diastasis. *J. Bone Joint Surg. 40-B:* 270, 1958.

Myhre, H. On osteochondritis dissecans trochleae tali. *Acta Radiol. 20:* 272, 1939.

Nagy, D. *Radiological Anatomy*, translated by A. Deak. Pergamon Press, New York, 1965.

Nancrede, C. B. Some new observations upon the anatomy and functions of the ankle and tibio-fibular joints. *Med Times*, p. 316, March 27, 1880.

Outland, T. Sprains and separations of the inferior tibiofibular joint without important fracture. *Am. J. Surg. (n.s.) 59:* 320, 1943.

Parsons, F. G. On the morphology of the tendo-Achillis. *J. Anat. Physiol. 28:* 414, 1894.

Paturet, G. *Traité d'anatomie humaine*. Masson et Cie, Paris, 1951.

Piersol, G. A., Ed. *Human Anatomy, Including Structure and Development and Practical Considerations*. J. B. Lippincott Company, Philadelphia, 1907.

Piersol, G. A. *Human Anatomy, Including Structure and Development and Practical Considerations*, ed. 8. J. B. Lippincott and Company, Philadelphia, 1923.

Quain's Elements of Anatomy, edited by W. Sharpey, A. Thomson, and J. Cleland, ed. 7, vol. 1. James Walton, London, 1867.

Quain's Elements of Anatomy, edited by E. A. Schäfer and G. D. Thane, ed. 10, vol. 2, part 2. Longmans, Green & Co., London, 1892.

Rauber's Lehrbuch der Anatomie des Menschen, edited by F. Kopsch, ed. 7, part 2. Verlag von Georg Thieme, Leipzig, 1906.

Rauber-Kopsch Lehrbuch und Atlas der Anatomie des Menschen, edited by W. Bargmann, H. Leonhardt, and G. Töndury, ed. 20, vol. 1. Georg Thieme Verlag, Stuttgart, 1968.

Ray, R. B., and Coughlin, E. J., Jr. Osteochondritis dissecans of the talus. *J. Bone Joint Surg. 29:* 697, 710, 1947.

Reck, W. Über die Verankerung der Achillessehne am Calcaneus beim Neugeborenen. *Anat. Anz. 128:* 281, 1971.

Rouvière, H. *Anatomie humaine, descriptive et topographique*, edited by G. Cordier and A. Delmas, ed. 9, vol. 3. Masson et Cie, Paris, 1962.

Rubin, G., and Witten, M. The talar-tilt angle and the fibular collateral ligaments: A method for the determination of talar tilt. *J. Bone Joint Surg. 42-A:* 311, 1960.

Ryker, N. J., Jr. *Glass Walkway Studies of Normal Subjects During Normal Level Walking*. Prosthetic Devices Research Project, Institute of Engineering Research, University of California, Berkeley. Series 11, issue 20. The Project, Berkeley, 1952.

Sammarco, G. J., Burstein, A. H., and Frankel, V. H. Biomechanics of the ankle: A kinematic study. *Orthop. Clin. North Am. 4:* 75, 1973.

Saunders, J. B. deC. M., Inman, V. T., and Eberhart, H. D. The major determinants in normal and pathological gait. *J. Bone Joint Surg. 35-A:* 543, 1953.

Schultz, A. H. Changes in fetuses due to formalin preservation. *Am. J. Phys. Anthropol. 2:* 35, 1919.

Sewell, R. B. S. A study of the astragalus. Part I. *J. Anat. Physiol. 38:* 233, 1904.

Shephard, E. Tarsal movements. *J. Bone Joint Surg. 33-B:* 258, 1951.

Simon, W. H. Scale effects in animal joints. II. Thickness and elasticity in the deformability of articular cartilage. *Arthritis Rheum. 14:* 493, 1971.

Simon, W. H., Friedenberg, S., and Richardson, S. Joint congruence: A correlation of joint congruence and thickness of articular cartilage in dogs. *J. Bone Joint Surg. 55-A:* 1614, 1973.

Smillie, I. S. *Osteochondritis Dissecans. Loose Bodies in Joints: Etiology, Pathology, Treatment*. E. & S. Livingstone, Edinburgh and London, 1960.

Smith, R. C. *Smith Total Ankle Surgical Procedure*. Wright Manufacturing Co. (411 North Third St., Memphis, Tenn. 38105), 1973.

Smith, R. C. Personal communication, 1974.

Sobotta, J. *Atlas of Descriptive Human Anatomy*, edited and translated by E. Uhlenhuth, ed. 7, vol. 1. Hafner, New York, 1957.

Staples, O. S. Ruptures of the fibular collateral ligaments of the ankle: Result study of immediate surgical treatment. *J. Bone Joint Surg. 57-A:* 101, 1975.

Steindler, A. The foot. Number 1. The pathomechanics of the static disabilities of foot and ankle. In *The American Academy of Orthopaedic Surgeons: Instructional Course Lectures*, edited by C. N. Pease, vol. 9. J. W. Edwards, Ann Arbor, 1952.

Steindler, A. *Kinesiology of the Human Body under Normal and Pathological Conditions*. Charles C Thomas Company, Springfield, Ill., 1955.

Swartling, R. D. *Tibial Torsion: A New Method for Measurement and the Change That Takes Place with Growth*. Biomechanics Laboratory, University of California, San Francisco and Berkeley. Technical Memorandum. The Laboratory, San Francisco, 1972.

Testut, L. *Traité d'anatomie humaine: Anatomie descriptive—histologie—développement*, ed. 3, vol. 1. Octave Doin, Editeur, Paris, 1896.

Testut, L., and Latarjet, A. *Traité d'anatomie humaine*, edited by A. Latarjet, ed. 9, vol. 1. G. Doin et Cie, Paris, 1948.

Todd, R. B., Ed. *The Cyclopaedia of Anatomy and Physiology*, edited by R. B. Todd, vol. 1. Longman, Brown, Green, Longmans, and Roberts, London, 1835–1836.

Toldt, C. *Anatomischer Atlas für Studierende und Ärzte*, ed. 8. Urban & Schwarzenberg, Berlin, 1914.

Wagner, W. F., Jr. Personal communication, 1974.

Weinert, C. R., Jr., McMaster, J. H., and Ferguson, R. J. Dynamic function of the human fibula. *Am. J. Anat. 138:* 145, 1973.

White, J. W. Torsion of the Achilles tendon: Its surgical significance. *Arch. Surg. 46:* 784, 1943.

Wiltse, L. L. Valgus deformity of the ankle: A sequel to acquired or congenital abnormalities of the fibula. *J. Bone Joint Surg. 54-A:* 595, 1972.

Winslow, Randolph. A reply to the article by Dr. C. B. Nancrede, of Phila., entitled "Some new observations upon the anatomy and functions of the ankle and tibio fibular joints." *Maryland Med. J. 7:* 28, 1880.

Wright, D. G., Desai, S. M., and Henderson, W. H. Action of the subtalar and ankle-joint complex during the stance phase of walking. *J. Bone Joint Surg. 46-A:* 361, 1964.

Wyller, Thomas. The axis of the ankle joint and its importance in subtalar arthrodesis. *Acta Orthop. Scand. 33:* 320, 1963.

INDEX